I0786979

Lose 44 Pounds (20kg) In 90 Days

My weight loss journey

How I lost 50 pounds (23 kgs) in 90 days and reversed my diabetes at the age of 62

Contents

Book Description

Have you been thinking of ways to lose weight? Do you wish to lose weight in 90 days so that you can improve your diabetes, feel younger and fitter like 20 years old? Are you wondering where to start?

If you answered "*Yes*" to these questions, then you have come to the right place!

When it comes to weight loss and improving your diabetes condition, it is best to have all your facts straight so that it does not take longer than it needs to be. Most people think that weight loss is just about appearance. The truth is, it is much more than that! Your weight affects many things in your life – self-esteem, health, quality of life, and mental and physical wellbeing.

Today, you must realize that achieving a healthy weight is something worth your time and effort. Here, I will share with you how I lost 50 pounds (23 KGs) in 90 days. My doctors kept increasing the diabetes doses, and soon they could have put me on insulin.

So, if you thought that weight loss is unattainable, let me show you how you can sustainably shed off those extra pounds, keep them off, and reverse your diabetes once and for all.

This is the time to embark on a weight loss journey to a slimmer, fitter, and healthier version of you. Today is the day to begin your transformation to a healthy weight loss. This book will help you understand that good-for-you weight loss has nothing to do with yo-yo dieting! You will understand that weight loss is a good way for your body to function well and empower you to achieve long-term success.

So, what are you still waiting for?

Come with me, and let's get started on a healthy weight loss journey with practical and healthy tips that will blow your mind.

Come with me!

Introduction

Weight loss has been a long-term issue for me, and when it inched up a couple of years, my type 2 diabetes became more unbearable. At one point in time, when the scale hit 255 pounds (115 kgs), I remember catching a glimpse of myself in the mirror, seeing this huge, fat person staring right back at me.

That was my eureka moment!

I immediately knew that if I didn't do something, my diabetes situation would worsen and eventually kill me. "Who will take care of my family when I'm gone? What will become of my wife and children? I can't allow my condition to take away all the resources they have left on my medication and eventually lose me to diabetes. I will not be able to rest in peace," I remember these racing through my mind – myriads and myriads of unanswered questions.

I started scanning through the internet for tips, guidebooks, anything I could find to improve my condition. Then I found one consultant in the South of India, and he guided me on how one can substantially lose weight and reverse diabetes. There, I knew that my weight was the best place to start. Weight loss marked the beginning of my journey to solving my type 2 diabetes condition.

What are you struggling with today? Are you overweight and struggling with type 2 diabetes as I was? Know that you can save yourself by working first on your weight. You must be willing to give up unhealthy lifestyle habits that are getting in your health.

You must understand that while doctors have known for years that weight loss can only prevent diabetes, the doctors kept pumping me with high doses, and soon they could have put me on insulin.

Type 2 diabetes occurs because of too much fat inside your liver and pancreas. Losing a significant amount of weight can kill off that fat so that your organs can begin to work well, and your insulin production will spring back to normal.

One common mistake I see people with type 2 diabetes is turning to the medication before they can have a chance to work on their weight. Weight loss is the first step for anyone that is first diagnosed with type 2 diabetes. The sooner you start working on losing those extra pounds, the better for you. Realize that while I managed to lose weight, people are different.

According to one study, 149 types 2 diabetes patients were assigned to a weight loss program, and another 149 were assigned to a treatment plan

with diabetes medications. Most of the research participants had been diagnosed with type 2 diabetes within the previous six years before the study. After 12 months, only 4% of the usual care patients had remission of diabetes.

Generally, remission in diabetes simply refers to one's blood sugar levels reverting to normal levels. The truth is, diabetes is not a one-and-done disease. There is always a chance that it could return if you don't pay attention to your weight or choose to go back to unhealthy habits.

While sugar is sweet, you must understand that taking too much of it might sour your health. If you load up on whole foods like grains, veggies, fruits, and dairy products, you give your body a supply of natural sugar, which the body digests slowly and ensures that the cells get a steady supply of energy. However, taking added sugars derived from processed foods and drinks poses a threat to your health.

According to the American Heart Association, you must not take over six teaspoons – roughly 25 grams – of added sugar per day if you are a woman and nine teaspoons – 36 grams – if you are a man.

Unfortunately, an average person takes way more than that – 22 teaspoons of sugar, which translates to 88 grams.

It is time to evaluate all your eating habits. What are you feeding your body?

In most cases, the biggest source of added sugar is Sugar-sweetened beverages. You must note that if you take soda every day and do not work out to trim the excess calories, the chances are that you will gain approximately 15 pounds in less than three years. Putting on excess weight is a recipe for diabetes and some types of cancers. Particularly, taking sugary drinks has the possibility of boosting your odds for type 2 diabetes. When there is excess sugar in the body, a signal is sent to make less insulin, which converts the food consumed into energy, or insulin fails to work at all.

You must note that when you work on losing even 10-15 pounds, that goes a long way in helping you manage your blood sugar levels. Unfortunately, most people blame salt for hypertension. However, researchers say that sugar is a more worrisome culprit for this condition. The way sugar is believed to raise the blood pressure levels is by making insulin levels spike above normal, making the blood vessels flexible and the kidneys prone to holding onto water and sodium.

Remember, taking a sugary diet irrespective of your body weight can raise LDL – the bad guys – cholesterol and lower HDL – the good guys – cholesterol. It also elevates the triglycerides' levels, hindering the proper work of enzymes responsible for breaking them down.

You are what you eat!

Read on to find out more!

Chapter 1 My weight loss journey

My weight loss journey is not so much of an overnight success story. The truth is, I did not have a magic pill that helped me lose weight. I did not eat a fad diet. Most people don't know that my weight loss journey was more of a roller coaster ride of trials, errors, and several milestones that eventually added to weight loss and a lifestyle change.

I was a very unhappy man trapped beneath baggy clothes and stretchy pants while also struggling with diabetes. Weight loss has been a long-term issue for me, and when it inched up a couple of years ago, my type 2 diabetes became more unbearable. When the scale hit 255 pounds, I remember catching a glimpse of myself in the mirror, seeing this huge, fat person staring right back at me.

Like I said earlier, this was my eureka moment!

That is when I knew that if I didn't do something, my diabetes situation would worsen and eventually kill me. "Who will take care of my family when I'm gone? What will become of my wife? I can't allow my condition to take away all the resources they have left on my medication and eventually lose me to diabetes. I will not be able to rest in peace," I remember these racing through my mind – myriads and myriads of unanswered questions.

My diabetes condition was getting worse, and the doctors kept pumping me with high doses, and soon they could have put me on insulin. I started reading on how best to deal with a situation like mine. That is when my desperation for weight loss inched up. I had no idea that my weight loss journey would turn into a journey of freedom, self-discovery, finding health, joy, and well-being.

I followed a very strict, no-carb diet with a very simple 6 stages diet each stage 14 days as suggested by my weight loss consultant. First, 14 days all I had was salads and proteins – veggies and boiled eggs. After that, at every stage, different foods like fish, meat, chicken, beans, etc. were added. There are no cheat days here. No alcohol. These are the things that played an important role in helping me lose weight fast and sustainably.

The other thing that helped me was 12-hours intermittent fasting during the night. What you must realize is that several resources on intermittent fasting available online are not trusted. Therefore, you have to find a plan that works best for you, which will help you achieve your weight loss goals.

My secret is simple – no-carb or low carb diet introduced at the different levels during the 90 days weight loss program and regular workouts!

I was never a fat boy as a child. I was very active in sports, played soccer and badminton, and won races at school. Those days, the only option you would eat was a homemade food that was fully fried and loaded with carbs. For us, food was food - we didn't know anything about carbs, fats, or proteins those days.

Things changed when I joined college and started drinking alcohol and indulging in greasy foods with a few friends. It got worse after college when I got into a sedentary lifestyle – no more sporting activities and traveling by bus. I had a more comfortable bike. Every day, I drank a few beers and ate restaurant food loaded with fatty oils and butter, which eventually saw me put on a lot of weight, especially on my belly.

I got married in 1983 to a very beautiful woman who, to date, has remained 45 kg (99 pounds). But did that stop my indulgence in food and alcohol? Not a chance! Before I knew it, five years into marriage and 255 pounds (115 kgs) up from 172 pounds (78 kgs).

My struggles and failures started!

I felt lethargic and tired all the time. People started calling me *motu, jadia* (Indian words for fat), and it hurt. People calling me names finally got to me and affected my self-esteem. In my forties, I could not handle my weight - breathlessness and slight pain in the knees.

I could take morning walks, hoping to lose weight only to give up after a few days. I signed up for gym membership and gave up after a few weeks. My waistline was now 48 inches, and finding clothes that could fit was a struggle because there was no plus size clothing in India then.

I tried eating less, going hungry, and drinking only tea for a few days at a stretch. It worked at first, and I few pounds only to gain it all back faster than it was gone. Soon, I was 50 years old. I was terrified because I knew that diabetes was hereditary, and it ran in my family.

My elder brother was diagnosed with diabetes at a very young age. It was uncontrollable as he indulged in starchy foods and drank alcohol more than I did. By the time he was 308 pounds (140 kgs), he had to undergo bariatric surgery. Both his kidneys got damaged, and now he is on dialysis three times a week. My father had diabetes, too but died at the age of 48 due to cardiac arrest.

I was living a very fearful life.

Each time I saw my elder brother's struggle, I knew my days were numbered. I knew I wasn't living; I was dying slowly. I had seen it all in my family. Every 1st January of the year, weight loss was my topmost new year's resolution, only to give up after the first few weeks.

Each time I consulted a dietician or nutritionist, they would give me a computer printout of a diet I needed to follow, but in vain! While I felt that I needed to change my lifestyle to live, some part of me didn't want to give up on the joy of drinking – beers, single malts, and wines.

On January 22nd, 2018, I celebrated my 60th birthday. I did my routine blood check-ups. My sugar levels fasting were at 190 and HBA1C at 8.9. My SGOT and SGPT also started to go haywire along with some other parameters. My doctor kept increasing the metformin dosage to control the blood sugar levels. Until then, no doctor had ever told me that diabetes could be reversed using diet. Every weight loss attempt failed, and the furthest I could go was 105 kgs (231 pounds) from 253 pounds (115 kgs).

Early 2019 I started coaching a young CEO of a technology company, and we met once a month. What shocked me was that though he was obese, he suddenly started losing weight. Between December 2019 and February 2020, he had lost around 20kg. That was a defining moment for me.

"Wow, 44 pounds (20 kgs) in 90 days, but how?" I asked
him. He said he had a consultant in Chennai in the south of
India.

He linked me up with his consultant, and I immediately got
in touch with him. I had seen the results and knew it was
THEN or NEVER. For me, that was the difference between
life and death. Having done comprehensive research on
weight loss in reversing diabetes, this consultant suggested
a very basic low carb diet plan, which explained what to eat
and what not to eat. I had to order loads of vitamins –
mostly online from the USA – which was a little expensive.
At first, it was scary taking lots of vitamins and
supplements. However, I knew this was the last chance I
had to make things right. The last thing I wanted was to get
in with doubts in mind.

March 15th, I started the program.

For the first 14 days, I only ate boiled eggs, Whey protein,
and salads coupled with a 12-hours intermittent fast at
night. In other words, if I had my dinner at 9 pm, I would
not eat anything until 9 am the following day. I started my
day with one TBS of cold-pressed coconut oil. I was eager
to see results, but the first seven days, nothing happened.

I got frustrated when I gained a little weight. I invited a
friend for breakfast, and I once again went back to my old

eating habits – 3 *Aloo parathas* (India bread stuffed with potatoes) with butter. I believed that diets didn't work. I had sleepless nights thinking about how I had failed and how my life was over. I knew diabetes would slowly take me to the grave, just like my brother and father did.

But after the weekend, my senses kicked in, and I called my consultant. I told him everything I felt and the Sunday breakfast I had with my friend. He sent me an explanation of how the body cells work and how they try to retain water before breakdown.

That was an eye-opener! I bought many books on intermittent fasting and keto diets to educate myself. As I read those books, I gained more and more insights into how weight loss works. I now understood the instructions clearly. I learned that the very first thing to do is get in the right mindset. Because of that, I wrote down my goals and affirmations on a small white card.

"My ideal weight is 165 pounds (75 kg) , and will live for 100+ years with great health."

I would affirm this every morning and at night before going to sleep, and you know what happened. My urge for alcohol went down, and each time I saw carbs or sweets, I did not have an urge for them.– not even a Single Malt in my home bar. I loved drinking on the weekends. It was all gone without any efforts. It was amazing how things magically changed. Amazing!

I also learned a vital 3 minutes of Nitric Oxide Dump exercise goes a long way. I have provided a youtube link of this particular exercise at the end of this book under resources. These 3 minutes of exercise in your bedroom every morning or night offers the benefit of a one-hour workout.

After a few days, my weight drastically dropped, and so did my blood sugar levels. Within 90 days, I had shed almost 50 pounds (23kgs). My fasting sugar levels dropped to below 106, and HBA1C went down to 5.90

Now, I am off all diabetes medications and am aiming to bring it down to 5.5. My energy levels are very high, and I am more productive, which has caused my income to increase significantly.

I have put my knowledge, experiences, and lessons in this book. I believe that if it worked for me, it's going to do for you—all the best during your journey. I would love to see you achieving your ideal weight within 90 days personally.

I have created a private Facebook group called "Weight Loss Achievers." The link is on the resources page at the end of the book.

Chapter 2 You are what you eat.

We have all heard the saying, "you are what you eat." But do we know what that means?

You must note that there is no such thing as a special diet exclusively for people with diabetes. While there is a wide range of ways to lose weight, there is no one-size-fits-all kind of diet. You must start by finding a way to eat fewer calories than you need.

The human body uses energy for everything it does – like breathing, working out, sleeping, and reading. Whenever you eat, you replace the energy used and hence maintain a healthy body weight. According to the health experts, it is recommended that a man consumes around 2,500 kcal/day to maintain healthy body weight, and women consume approximately 2,000 kcal/day.

However, some people require different amounts of calories depending on the kind of work, how active they are, and their health management goals. The key is for you to find a plan you enjoy, and that fits in perfectly well with your daily routine/lifestyle. We are all different from each other, and what works for you may not work for others.

What are you feeding your body with? Are you giving it too many calories than it needs?

Most packaged foods, drinks, or snacks are loaded with fructose, a simple sugar in veggies and fruits. The liver turns that into fat for storage. This means that regularly pumping your body with fructose promotes a buildup of tiny fat droplets in the liver – otherwise referred to as non-alcoholic fatty liver disease. If you choose to make an early diet change, this can be reversed. However, over time, there will be swelling and scarring of the liver causing damage.

The more you load up on sugars, the more you promote tooth decay. This is because what you eat feeds the bacteria in the mouth, leaving behind acid that wears away the tooth enamel. Some of the common offenders are dried fruits, sugary drinks, chocolates, candy, and others. The truth is, these foods are almost as acidic as battery acid! It is not bad to indulge from time to time, but when you do, ensure that you at least rinse the mouth with water or milk afterward to neutralize the acidity.

Additionally, pumping your body with sugars during the day has been shown to mess with your blood glucose levels, causing a spike and crash of energy. Taking a bowl of ice cream in the evening risks keeping you awake throughout the night or shortening the time you are in a deep sleep, making it impossible to get up feeling refreshed. According to new research, the insulin-producing cells are not dead but inactive in type 2 diabetes. Putting a type 2 diabetes patient on a diet can do marvelous things to their beta cells.

In other words, lifestyle changes like weight loss and workout regimes have been shown to have a large impact on diabetes. Once you are diagnosed with type 2 diabetes, you must immediately get on a weight loss program to turn it around. Studies show that taking 3-month diet trials and lifestyle changes before medication works wonders. It worked for me, and it most certainly will work for you.

Often, patients who are newly diagnosed with diabetes see their sugars melt back to normal ranges after working on losing excess body weight and making other lifestyle modifications. While this is good news, you must bear in mind that effort is not everything. Once you rise that high, there is a high chance of your sugar rising again. In that case, weight management is critically important and worth it. It helps to keep to a very low-carb diet.

Getting in the right mindset

One thing you must note is that the pros and cons accompany every weight loss strategy. However, for you to work through it, you must get in the right mindset. You must achieve your goal first in the mind before you can make it a reality.

Shifting your mindset for weight loss is one of the keys to losing weight. Realize that you cannot change your weight from the outside before you get your inner resolve and intention aligned with your goals. Most people try to lose weight by wanting to "fix" themselves. This mentality makes them jump into exercise ad diet plans out of self-deprecation while they still call themselves "fat" and feel less than they are all together.

Losing weight is not about focusing the mind on quick fixes. It is setting the mind on sustainability and wellbeing. Your mindset should be that you are doing this to improve your health, enjoyment, and longer life.

A negative mindset is a recipe for failure.

Here's what will help you adopt a positive mindset;

Be honest with yourself.

Losing weight requires that you accept the painful truth – why you are overweight or obese. It's okay to come to terms with the truth so that you can change unhealthy habits. Take a minute to reflect on what is true for you. Are you pumping your body with fast foods, sodas, and sweets?

Are you living a sedentary lifestyle? Is there an underlying condition contributing to your weight gain?

While it may seem silly to accept something painful, the truth is that it is the first step to helping you get in the right mindset for successful weight loss.

Whatever it is that is causing you to put on weight, realize that it can be controlled. Even if you have an underlying condition, you can safely lose weight. Start by talking to your doctor about it to determine the best approach to losing weight.

Once you know you are in control of your weight, you can only believe you will eventually realize your weight loss goals.

Visualize what you want

Why do you want to lose weight? Is it to eliminate a pre-existing health condition like diabetes? Do you want to get back in shape and feel confident again?

Whatever your reasons, let that be your motivation each day. Visualize what you want and what your life will be like once you achieve your goal. What helped me most was creating a vision board for my weight loss journey. Each morning I woke up, and before retiring to bed, I revisited my vision board as a source of motivation to keep working at it.

Use affirmations

Each day, remind yourself how capable and incredible you are. Remind yourself that you can achieve anything you set your mind to. Tell yourself that every day. Affirmations play a significant role in helping you get in the right weight loss mindset. Some of the affirmations that helped me get in a positive mindset include eating to nourish my wellbeing. I am in charge of what I put in my mouth and how much I get into my body. Every day, I am getting fitter, healthier, and more confident. Working out makes me feel good about myself. I am committed to taking care of myself by adopting healthy habits. My body craves healthy foods. Every day, I am losing weight. I am a weight loss success story. I am going to live for 100+ years with great health.

Adopting a negative mindset when you have goals to achieve will not get you anywhere. However, a positive mindset is contagious. Turn those negative thoughts around and start making positive affirmations about your health, goals, and overall wellbeing.

At first, you might think that it is ridiculous to just say things that are obvious to you is untrue. However, once you start making positive affirmations about your weight loss, the truth will begin unfolding.

Quit comparing

When you first start your weight loss journey, you may feel envious of those looking their best. But what you don't know is that some of those people had to work hard to get that body. Don't look at people who are at the end of their weight loss journey and compare yourself to them. If you do, you will be discouraged. Instead, use them as a motivation that weight loss is indeed achievable.

Remind yourself that everyone who has achieved their weight loss goals has to start by learning how to eat a **healthy** diet, work out, and do intermittent fasting – and you can too!

We all have our journey and story – and now is the time you write yours too.

Be patient

When you are impatient, it is easy to lose sight of your weight loss goals. At some point during your weight loss journey, you might feel like your mindset has shifted, and you are no longer as focused as you were when you first got started.

What you must understand is that weight loss is not something that happens overnight. You must exercise patience, consistency, and keep working at it. When you maintain consistency, the chances are that you will achieve weight loss, build a strong, healthy habit, and keep that weight off in the long-term.

The last thing you want is to lose weight only to go back to your old habits and gain it all back. Remind yourself that each passing day draws you closer to your goal. Your part is to make each day count and have some progress to show of it.

Read on to learn some of the mistakes I made during the first months of weight loss. You want to read this to avoid them and achieve your weight loss and **reverse** your diabetes as soon as possible.

Chapter 3 Mistakes I made during the first months of weight loss.

The very first month of my weight loss journey was characterized by hopes, challenges, questions, obstacles, and accomplishments. There were times when I made mistakes. The truth is, however, prepared and motivated you might be; there will always be days when you feel like you can't get things right.

It could be that unintentional sugar binge, unrealistic goals, skipped workouts, or something else. Whatever it is, you must understand that bumps and obstacles are part of the journey. The key here is for you to find the right detour and creative solutions that will help you keep moving in the right direction without allowing these obstacles to derail your weight loss goals.

Here are some of the mistakes I made;

Forcing yourself to eat foods you hate

How many people have you heard are on a diet? Of those people, how many of them have been successful at keeping it sustainable?

The main reason most diet plans fail is that we chose something that is not sustainable in the first place. You cannot force yourself to eat something you cannot stand just because you are on a prescribed diet plan. Trust me; if you do, you will not keep it on track in the long-term. You need to understand that when you treat your diet in this way, you turn it into a form of punishment, which rarely works. Punishing yourself by eating something you can't stand makes it easy to justify a high-calorie diet as a treat, hence undermining your efforts.

Most people don't realize that when they force themselves to eat foods in the name of healthy eating, you risk hating foods in that group by mere association. If you dislike kale by forcing yourself to keep adding it in your diet plan, you might hate all leafy greens.

The best trick is to look for more palatable alternatives. There are many foods to choose from in a group if you don't like one or two. If you hate kale, why not consider swiss chard, baby spinach, or arugula instead? The key is to keep an open mind and allow yourself to learn what foods help you achieve your goals without compromising on your palate. This way, you position yourself to develop lifelong healthy habits that will help you improve your health.

Weighing myself too often

When you embark on a weight loss journey, you may find it counterintuitive to keep off looking at the scale. One thing I didn't understand at first was why my weight was fluctuating every day. I kept on checking the scale every day, and when I noticed an increase in weight, I felt demoralized. I felt like quitting – and I did from time to time.

It is important to note that your weight will fluctuate for a wide range of reasons – like hormonal changes and water retention when you are on a weight loss journey. To avoid getting discouraged and risk calling it quits, it is best if you weigh yourself only once every week at the same time – or maybe don't do it at all. You can choose to take circumference measurements instead, like your waist and hips. These metrics play a significant role in serving as indicators of overall health and success.

Try as much as you can not get caught up in the numbers. It is best if you find your meaningful why and stick to it. Constantly remind yourself why you started this weight loss journey in the first place. Remind yourself how much you want to reverse your diabetes and improve your overall quality of life and not just the arbitrary numbers on the scale. When you have more energy to keep up the exercises and improve your health, it is way meaningful than just numbers on the scale.

Testing the waters

After a couple of weeks of sticking to the weight loss plan, you may be tempted to indulge in some of your old food vices. When you yield to this temptation, it becomes difficult to keep off the bad behaviors you have worked so hard over the last couple of weeks. However, if your newfound sense of self-confidence bolsters you, it seems more manageable than ever.

Testing the waters is a set up for mental punishment, and that is the last thing you want to put yourself through.

Wanting to eat cookies or ice cream just to prove that they don't control, you will only set you up in guilt after eating it and puts the reins tighter on your workouts and meal plans.

Simply stick to your plan and only indulge once in a blue moon.

Aiming "perfect" eating

It is great to have discipline and motivation. However, when you slip into the "all-or-nothing" mentality, it can mess up your weight loss journey and make it impossible for you to improve your diabetes.

The best thing you can do here is to steer clear of overly rigid diet like steamed asparagus, only eating grilled chicken, or allowing a zero indulgence. Realize that no one is perfect, and you if you aim for perfection, you might risk extreme burnouts that will only make your healthy lifestyle short-lived.

I encourage you to create a list of all the foods you consider non-negotiable. Take a minute to reflect on all the foods you love most and not imagine giving upon them. Suppose you don't consider all the foods you like as non-negotiables. In that case, the chances are that you will stir up extra anxiety when those foods are not included, even if in small quantities into your diet to make it enjoyable the whole process successful.

Skimping on sleep

Before you start patting yourself on the back or chest-beating for prepping meals into the wee hours of the night and getting up at down to work out while feeling drowsy, realize that insufficient sleep will sabotage your weight loss goals. According to experts, adults who sleep less than 7 hours a night are at a 30-80% risk of developing type 2 diabetes, cardiovascular disease, and hypertension compared to those who get 8 hours of sleep.

According to research, a lack of sleep is often a potential risk for weight gain and the growing obesity epidemic. This is mainly because it disrupts a wide range of hormonal and metabolic processes. Another study also reveals that sleep deprivation contributes to increased appetite because a change in sleep patterns alters the hormones responsible for regulating hunger.

To ensure your weight loss efforts remain on track and support your overall wellbeing, you must devote at least eight solid hours of good quality sleep.

Accepting imposters

Have you ever thought about why food manufacturers remove fat, gluten, and sugar from their products? They want you to believe that you have the very best of both worlds – the wonderful tastes you love minus the guilt. Most people don't see that those ingredients are almost always replaced with other ones that are bad or even worse than the ones removed!

Let us consider an example where fat is removed but is replaced with excess sugars, or sugar is removed and replaced with artificial ingredients, or gluten is replaced with refined carbs.

Do you see what is happening here?

The best thing is for you to choose options naturally free from ingredients you wish to steer clear of. For instance, you can choose to try naturally occurring gluten-free quinoa instead of ones filled with pasta. This way, you still enjoy the taste while ensuring that you consume something that is nutrient-rich.

Eating (or drinking) too much fruit

Even though fruits are healthy alternatives to cookies, cakes, and favorite packaged snacks, you must note that you will have difficulties shedding off the excess weight if you consume them daily. Even though they are natural, you must note that it is pure sugar. If you are not working out hard enough, excess sugar will be stored away as fat.

Unfortunately, most people think that by switching from sodas to fruit juices, they make it better to achieve weight loss and improve their health and overall wellbeing. The truth is, fruit juices are 100% sugar. They don't have fiber or water to slow down the process of digestion. They also have the same caloric content as a glass of soda. Whenever you are not sure of something, simply reach for water.

Overestimating the power of exercise

For optimal fitness, heart health, improved mood, and higher energy levels, exercise remains the key element. However, you must not assume that those killer workouts give you a free pass to pump your body with whatever you please.

You have to realize that even the most rigorous workouts call for a slight bump in your caloric intake. Those calories must be derived from nutritious foods that will fuel the body and recover.

A common mistake we make is focusing too much on cardio workouts. Even though cardio activities burn calories and improve your heart health, energy levels, and lung capacity, it should never be your sole exercise. When you rely on cardio alone, you burn not only fat but also muscle. Losing muscle mass causes a slowed metabolism giving you a softer and rounder shape. Remember, you want to lose weight and keep it off – and the best way to achieve that is through strength training, which maintains and builds muscle mass.

Not giving the brain time to adjust.

For most people, it is easy to get trapped in the physical aspects of weight loss. However, the most important question you must ask yourself is how your mental game is like.

Your brain needs a sufficient amount of time to reset and adjust to your new diet plan. When you change your meal plan, your brain will try to fight back because it does not find it satisfying at first.

If your brain is used to certain tastes – like fatty foods, salts, high fructose corn syrups, and others – it will take a long time for you to adjust mentally to a plant-based diet, for example. The best trick is to do it gradually so that the brain does not fight you so much. With time, the brain will learn to accept it, and your new diet will become normal.

Ignoring portion sizes

At first, I was always tempted to fill my plate with healthy-boosting superfoods. What I did not realize is that while food is healthy, portion sizes also matters. When you purpose to consume reasonable portions of your diet, you will fill up with a variety of nutrients your body needs.

Realize that nutritious foods like walnuts, dark chocolates, almonds, red wine, and avocados are loaded with calories. Even taking berries alone can add up to an excess of sugars when consumed with reckless abandon. It is great to carefully choose your superfoods using common sense as far as portion sizes are concerned.

Ignoring feelings of hunger.

Did you know that your body has a built-in mechanism that regulates food intake?

Unfortunately, most of us ignore this completely!

Humans are conditioned to drink and eat at social events where there is tremendous peer pressure, making it challenging for people on a weight loss program. Learning to pay attention to hunger cues will help you eat exactly what you need and nothing more.

Each time you are tempted to clean your plate or reach out for a snack, you first need to ask yourself whether you are hungry. Is your appetite response to stress, time of say, boredom, or peer pressure? If you are hungry – truly – then go ahead and eat. If not, just don't! If you are hungry, only ensure that you eat what you need, and once you feel satisfied, stop.

This is one of the hardest parts of beginning a new diet plan. The truth is, hunger is only a determinant of when you need to eat, and when you allow yourself to feel hungry, only then is eating more satisfying.

That said, all these are mistakes I made when I first started my weight loss journey. If you pay attention to them, you will strategically position yourself to make better choices to avoid disappointments, unnecessary temptations, and frustrations. Realize that no weight loss journey is free of ups and downs. Therefore, ensure that you tailor your diet and workout plan to the things you like, needs, goals, and avoid things you dislike. This way, you can constantly move in the right direction and attain success.

Chapter 4 Benefits of weight loss

We all want to lose weight for a wide range of reasons, and no matter what your reason may be, there are several changes you will enjoy on the inside and outside. Your confidence will grow on the outside, but several transformations happen on the inside. Here are some of the benefits you will enjoy on your weight loss journey;

Psychological benefits

Some of the things you will notice when you lose weight are the physical changes that occur. Your body gets healthier, and your chances of developing such diseases as cancer, heart disease, type 2 diabetes, and brain diseases decline significantly.

Unfortunately, most people do not stop to appreciate all the psychological benefits that losing weight brings. You must understand that besides getting healthier in the physical sense, there are positive transformations that happen on the mental side of your wellbeing. These mental changes are very important too, and they will help you embrace your new self in a positive, healthy, and productive way possible.

Remember that positive changes do not just happen on the physical and mental way of thinking. According to research studies, evidence shows that when one feels better about themselves, their self-esteem, quality of life, and body image improve a great deal. All these things happen because you have started eating healthy – and is why you must strive to lose weight.

As you begin to travel your weight loss journey, you must not lose sight of the bigger picture because that offers a wholesome understanding of the impact of eight loss. You are not just losing weight. You must feel good in your new body and have the drive to maintain it well.

Here are some of the psychological benefits of weight loss;

Improved self-esteem

According to research, studies show that when you lose weight, your sense of self-esteem improves. Changing your eating habits/patterns to healthier food choices and exercising, you are improving your physical body, and these changes make you start feeling good about your new self. The truth is, the more weight you lose, the more your self-esteem grows.

A decline in depressive symptoms

Out of over 17 studies, the only one did not see a change in the depressive symptoms that accompanies weight loss. Most of the people on a weight loss program reported feeling much better when they lost weight. They no longer had feelings of anxiety and depressions because they became more comfortable in their new bodies.

According to my physical therapist, the initial motivation to hit the gym and keep the habit going might be to lose weight at first. However, as you keep at it, the routine begins to boost your mood and a kick of self-confidence.

Realize that, when your body is under stress – climbing the stairs – the brain is stimulated to release endorphins that serve as painkillers that help relieve the discomfort you are feeling at that moment. These endorphins have also been shown to have power in the brain to generate feelings of euphoria.

It's time to take up a challenge and begin working out.

The next time you are at the gym, use these mood-lifting workouts;

If you feel a little down, simply try the upward dog. According to a study published in the Journal of Alternative and complementary medicine (2010), the anxiety and mood levels of people who practiced yoga for at least an hour three times a week found that this exercise was associated with an increase in GABA levels. This is an amino acid and neurotransmitter that plays a significant role in lowering anxiety.

Additionally, people who practiced deep yogic breathing experienced an increase in the flow of oxygen, which contributed to the proper functioning of body organs, including the brain. All these promoted an overall improvement in the mood because it simply subjects the parasympathetic nervous system into high gear, promoting relaxation.

If you are new to yoga, the first thing you need to do is learn how to breathe correctly. Simply breathe in through your nose and count to five. Hold your breath for at least two counts and then exhale through the nose to five. This ensures that the lungs are completely emptied.

Repeat this practice at least five times.

Once you are done, you are ready to merge the breathing with body movements. You can practice at home or seek a yoga instructor's help for a session of an hour per week. That said, if you choose to do this even just for 15 minutes every day, you can improve your outlook and mood greatly. The secret here is consistency.

Pilates

Your mood can be greatly affected by your sleep problems. One thing you must realize is that good sleep is impossible to achieve is you are stressed. It just makes it hard to wind down. However, all is not lost because there is a promising fix for that. A study published by Appalachian State University reported that practicing Pilates is linked with better sleep and, in effect, helps boost mood.

Research participants who did Pilates on a mat for 75 or 50 minutes at least twice or thrice a week have a lower likelihood of experiencing trouble during sleep. The improvement in sleep is accompanied by increased bodily awareness. When you are in sync with yourself, you are less likely to experience stress, hence enjoy relaxation and good moods.

To practice Pilates, you can take mat classes at the gym for at least an hour. To enjoy results soon, do this at least three times a week.

Most people think that cycling is just about spinning the wheels. The truth is when you are spinning the wheels, you get a boost of energy, according to researchers at the University of Georgia, Athens. During cycling, the brain experiences positive electrical changes by activating the neural circuits that help one feel energized. Physical activity is not tiring; it is stimulating and energizing.

The next time you are working out at the gym, try cycling on a stationary bike for at least 15 minutes three times a week. You will not only lose weight but also consistently enjoy a boost in energy levels. Also, don't limit your cycling sessions to just the gym. Studies show that cycling outdoors does not only boost energy levels but also help lower feelings of anxiety and depression, hence boosting your moods.

Weight lifting

One thing we know for sure is that lifting dumbbells is great for toning the triceps. However, you need to understand that this is also a great exercise for toning mental muscles. A study published in the Journal of Clinical and Experimental Neuropsychology revealed that older adults who engaged in low-intensity weight training exercises at least 3-5 times a week for one month had an improved cognitive ability compared to those who did not practice weight training.

They had an improved ability to plan, multitask, and regulate behaviors. In other words, weight training plays an important role in boosting one's attention span, promoting their ability to make the right choices even on challenging brain tests. These workouts boost the participant's overall mood by strengthening the muscle connection in the brain and the generation of new neurons that promote the flexibility of existing neurons.

Tai chi

Tai chi has been reported as a stress-busting workout that combines positions and movements that flow into each other. Traditionally, this workout is done in a standing position, and your role is to repeatedly shift your weight back and forth. As you do this, your lower and upper body muscles are actively engaged, and you also engage in rhythmic breathing. Considering that these shifts are slow and fluid, the muscles tend to relax better, the minds clams down, and your balance, strength, and flexibility are improved.

It is a meditation in motion!

It is known to stimulate the body's flow – commonly referred to as Chi in Chinese, which means life force.

Each time you practice Tai Chi, your precise actions focus the mind on what matters most and reminds you to take things slow, boosting your overall mood and feeling about yourself.

Nitric Oxide Release Workout

This is my favorite

The nitric oxide dump is a new version of high-intensity interval training (HIIT) developed by Dr. Zach Bush. This approach was mainly designed to stimulate nitric oxide release, which can catalyze and promote health.

The primary role of nitric oxide is that it lines the inner layer of your blood vessels, the endothelium, and acts as a messenger molecule that transmits signals to cells in various parts of your body – like the cardiovascular, nervous, and immune systems.

During exercise, nitric oxide is released, and then it works its way into the smooth muscles, causing them to relax. You must note that nitric oxide Dump uses simple movements done in quick succession. This offers similar benefits to longer workouts, except that in this case, they are accomplished in just a short time. According to Dr. Bush, it is one of the best ways to tone your body's systems.

The good thing with the Nitric Oxide Dump is that it uses up just a fraction of your time, with a single session lasting between three to four minutes. Considering this technique is ideally repeated three times a day, you eventually use around 15 minutes.

This is another simple exercise you can engage in to enhance your endurance and strength. This exercise should be performed at least once a week and increase the frequency as your strength grows.

The trick here is to tighten your core, stabilize your glutes as you lift weights. You must pay attention to your posture to keep it upright. What matters most is how you walk with the weight. When setting the weights down, ensure that your core is as tight as possible. The two ways to perform this is to focus on time and distance. Typically, 100 feet is sufficient enough for a cumbersome carry.

Farmer's walk acts to stabilize the body, increase the forearm muscles, and improve your wrist and hands' grip strength. It also boosts your mobility.

What happens if you overdo it?

The chances are that you will cause muscle strain and likely result in injury. Even as you work on losing weight, you must pay attention to maintaining your body's balance even as you work on increasing your body's ability to shed off extra weight.

Body Image

This is self-explanatory. When you work on losing weight, your body consistently improved, and so does your body image. Your level of dissatisfaction often measures body image and how high you rate your body – body shape, looks, esteem, etc. – on a scale of 1 to 10. As you start enjoying an improvement in your body image, you become more motivated to achieve your weight loss goals and maintain a healthy body in the long term.

Generally, when you lose weight, your satisfaction in your body and appearance grows. You start to feel good about yourself and enjoy a healthy and quality life. The most important thing is that you stick to changes in your eating habits to keep enjoying the results of weight loss.

Health benefits

Lowering the risk of heart disease

Losing weight plays an important role in lowering the risk of heart disease. This is mainly because it lowers the blood levels of LDL (Low-density lipoproteins) while raising high-density lipoproteins levels. In other words, you get more of the good stuff and less of the bad stuff.

You are wondering, how can I boost my levels of good cholesterol naturally?

The best tricks to help you naturally boost your HDL levels is to;

Get active at least half-hour every day, doing moderate to high-intensity workouts.

Choose good fats – mono- and poly-unsaturated fats commonly found in plants, fish, tuna, salmon, and nuts. When you eat, ensure that you pay attention to your portion sizes and keep them small.

Quit smoking and drinking.

Maintain or lower blood sugar levels

According to research, type 2 diabetes has been associated with obesity. However, it is evident that when you lose weight, you stand a chance of lessening or even reversing its effects. One study shows that type 2 diabetes patients do not depend on their blood sugar-regulating medications once they lose weight. In other words, with an aggressive weight loss plan, these patients managed to lower their medication requirements fast. Their blood glucose levels improved, and so did their diabetes markers. In extreme cases, patients can discontinue their insulin medication.

Build stronger bones and joints

When you are obese or overweight, your body exerts so much pressure on the weight-bearing joints around the hips, lower back, and knees. This causes wear and tear of the protective cartilages around the joints leading to osteoarthritis, characterized by pain, loss of mobility, and stiffness. According to researchers, weight loss lowers the risk and progression of osteoarthritis.

When you work on shedding off several pounds, you increase the body's ability to tolerate more activity and impact. Imagine training for a half-marathon without all the aches and pain – isn't that incredible? You can now do all those weight-bearing workouts while also increasing your bone density. This means stronger bones with every move you make. All this and more are within reach once you shed off those extra pounds.

Clearer, glowing and youthful skin

When you are constantly pumping your body with processed foods, sweets, and all the world's calories, it all shows up on your skin. Research demonstrates that high blood sugar levels are associated with skin breakouts and premature aging – otherwise referred to as glycation.

The truth is, sugar molecules attach to collagen and cause hardening and breakage of collagen. This results in wrinkling and premature aging. Therefore, cleaning up your diet for weight loss is not just the goal, but also helps lower the signs of aging skin.

Better sleep

According to WHO, obesity has reached epidemic proportions globally, with at least 2.8 million people dying each year due to being overweight or obese. Once associated with high-income countries, obesity is now also prevalent in low- and middle-income countries.

 One study of 250 obese with type 2 diabetes research participants were divided into two groups. One of the groups went through an extensive weight loss program comprising of exercises and controlled diets. In contrast, the other went through informational sessions aimed at promoting proper maintenance of diabetes.

The results?

Well, let's just say that the weight loss group shed off at least 24 pounds, and surprisingly, a good number of them improved their sleep significantly.

Improved sex drive

As discussed earlier, weight loss is often accompanied by a boost in confidence. This goes a long way in giving you that sex life you have been dying for. Research at the University of Pennsylvania School of Medicine reveals that women who went through a weight loss program for a year lost at least 32.7% of their original weight. Their sex drive, lubrication, arousal, and sexual satisfaction were over the roof.

Reduced risk of breast cancer

Research studies show that losing even just 5% of your original weight lowers breast cancer risk. At least 400 overweight and obese women were grouped into 4; those who engage in exercises only, diets only, both diet and exercise, and the control group who did not change their diet and exercise habits.

This study's results were surprising – increased estrogen levels, especially for women who focused on changing their diets and workout routines.

Chapter 5 Why diabetics struggle with weight loss

According to research, about 90% of people with type 2 diabetes are either obese or overweight. One thing you must note is that while obesity is a major contributing factor to the development of diabetes, the greatest driver is the high levels of insulin.

If you are wondering why people with diabetes struggle with weight loss, here are some reasons to gain a deeper insight;

High insulin levels and insulin is a fat-storage hormone.

We all have glucose in our blood at all times. It is the source of energy that largely is derived from carbohydrates. In other words, when you consume carbs, your blood sugar levels rise.

Insulin is a hormone produced by the pancreas. One of the functions of insulin is to help get glucose out of the blood and into cells. For this to happen, insulin levels have to rise along with the rise in glucose levels. For instance, when you eat a high carb diet, the glucose levels in the blood rise, causing a rise in insulin levels. Once it gets to the cells, it is used for energy.

For someone with type 2 diabetes, this process does not work well!

In other words, your body has developed resistance to insulin signals. This means that insulin is not as effective at moving glucose out of the blood and into the cells as it should be. This way, you end up with elevated glucose levels in the blood after eating a carb diet, which is chronically dangerous.

The body responds to this by making more insulin to get the job done. Remember, insulin has many other functions other than the regulation of blood glucose levels. It works by promoting fat storage, hence blocking the release of fat from fat storages in the body. Therefore, instead of losing weight, you keep putting on more weight – thanks to all that insulin!

Recommended eating patterns often fail by keeping you hungry even when your blood sugar is high

Most people with type 2 diabetes are told to eat carbs but ensure that the overall calories they get are fewer. We are told to eat small portions throughout the day to help keep the blood sugar levels steady.

Unfortunately, we find that we are hungry most of the time, always thinking about food or craving something to eat. The truth is, this is a survival instinct at work that even those with a strong will find it challenging to withstand. In other words, your psychology is fighting you. What is worse is that the small portions with carbs often cause a spike in the blood sugar levels, followed by a sharp drop that brings a roller coaster of feelings that stimulate hunger.

This makes it hard to lose weight!

Type 2 diabetes medications often drive weight gain.

Do you recall that your body's insulin is a fat-storage hormone?

This also applies to the insulin prescription you have been given – whether given through an injection or a pump. This explains why a commonly prescribed insulin often ends up in weight gain.

Another drug used for the treatment of type 2 diabetes – Sulfonylureas – is known to stimulate the pancreas to produce insulin. This means that high levels of insulin in circulation means more fat storage, which results in one putting on more weight.

So, what is the solution to all these challenges?

One thing you must understand is that people with type 2 diabetes are insulin resistant. This simply means that their tissues do not respond as they should to insulin. Remember that insulin is supposed to move glucose from the blood into cells for energy. If the body cannot respond to insulin, then your blood glucose levels will remain chronically high. The direct solution here is to lower the source of high blood sugar itself, which is carb intake.

In most cases, insulin resistance is termed "carb intolerance" mainly because when you are insulin resistant and then consume carbs, your blood sugar levels will not be lowered effectively. Therefore, by consuming fewer carbs, you lower glucose levels in circulation and insulin secretion.

Realize that nutritional ketosis, a natural metabolic state of the body burning fat for energy instead of carbs as the primary fuel, can also reverse diabetes. Unlike in the case of carb intake, fat intake does not trigger a spike in blood sugar levels. This makes fats a better source of fuel for anyone with insulin resistance.

According to research studies, type 2 diabetes patients lose at least 12% of their starting weight in less than six months when they use nutritional ketosis.

Chapter 6 Weight Loss Challenge

One of the most critical parts of making a lifestyle changing is deciding to do it!

An excellent place to start your weight loss journey is to challenge yourself. You must work hard to look great. Your weight loss challenge aims at testing you mentally and physically. You must be dedicated to working towards your goals. Trust me; the results will be worth it.

In this chapter, we will have a 14-day warm-up challenge that will help you focus on losing weight, improving your health, and staying fit. With this challenge, you will lose weight and gain strength and confidence to maintain a healthy lifestyle.

Remember, mindset is critical, ensuring you achieve success. You can do anything you put your mind to. Once you manage this 14-day challenge, you must ensure that you keep working at it until you achieve your goals. In other words, you must eat right and workout regularly. Bear in mind that a healthy lifestyle is a permanent change. You are not just doing this as a temporary phase.

These exercises work perfectly well by engaging them for 45 seconds and taking 15 seconds to rest in between. If you can complete each of the routines at least three times and then take a minute to rest, you will have completed a circuit. Exercises will help burn calories and change your mindset. By working out every day, you are training yourself to get better and make healthier choices.

Matching your diet with workouts will help you get consistent results.

So, are you ready to start your weight loss challenge? Come with me!

Here are some of the exercises you will do on your challenge;

Plyo-push up: simply start on the floor in a palm plank and then push into your palms so that your body explodes off the floor. Ensure that your feet are firmly planted on the floor at all times. Then land in a start position with your elbows soft and relaxed.

Speed skater Lunge

In a standing position, start jumping right foot to the right, bend the left leg, and then cross it behind the right one to land in a deep lunge with your right leg slightly bent at a right angle. Reach your left arm across your body to touch the floor at the front of your right toe. Then switch sides to jump left foot to the left and repeat the same.

High-Knees sprint

Begin to run in place and pull your knees towards your chest and vigorously bend your arms.

Pilates teaser

Start by lying faceup on the floor. Slightly bend your knees over the hips and arms extended up with palms facing each other. Roll your upper body and then extend your legs to get in a sitting position such that the body forms a V shape, and your arms are parallel to the legs. Pause there for a minute before rolling your upper body back down. Do this one vertebra after the other while your legs are still in the air. Once your shoulders rest on the floor, return to your starting position.

Burpee

From a standing position, crouch and plant your palms on the ground. Jump your feet back to plan while ensuring your abs remain tight. Slowly lower your chest and thighs on the floor. Press up to plank and begin to jump your feet towards your hands. It's okay if you can't get that high at the beginning. But as you keep working at it, try to jump as high as you can.

Jump-switch Lunge

In a standing position, lunge forward using your left foot and bend your knee at 90 degrees. Then jump as high as you can, swinging your arms overhead and switch legs in the air. As you land, ensure your arms are on your sides, and your right foot is forward – and bend your knee immediately. Alternate to the right foot and repeat the same.

Squat jack

Starting on a standing position, drop into a squat position, and bring your fists in front of your chest with your elbows bent on the sides. Jump with your feet wide, straight your legs, swing arms out to your sides and up such that they meet overhead.

14-days challenge

Days of the week	Challenge
Day 1	20 High-Knee Sprints Keep Portions In Check Keep Grains in Check
Day 2	20 Jump-Switch Lunges Eat Only When Hungry

	Downsize Your Dinnerware
Day 3	20 Squat Jacks Go for a Walk Bust Out the Scale
Day 4	20 Burpees Never Skip Breakfast Reduce Sodium
Day 5	20 Speed Skater Lunges Say No to Junk Food
Day 6	20 Pilates Teasers Nix Processed Foods
Day 7	20 Jump-Switch Lunges Track Total Calories Eat Only When Hungry

Day 8	20 Plyo Push-Ups Shop for Whole Foods Sleep 8+ Hours
Day 9	30 High-Knee Sprints Meal Prep Cut 100 Calories
Day 10	30 Burpees Ramp Up Protein Intake
Day 11	30 Squat Jacks Keep a Food Journal
Day 12	30 Speed Skater Lunges Put Veggies or Fruit on Every Plate
Day 13	30 Pilates Teasers

	Know Your Healthy Fats Eliminate Distractions
Day 14	30 Jump-Switch Lunges Reorganize Your Pantry/Fridge Eat at the Table

Chapter 7 Steps for Weight Loss Success for People with Type 2 Diabetes

While losing weight is at the top of most people's to-do lists, the truth is that this is especially important for those who have type 2 diabetes. When you carry excess body fat, you increase your body's resistance to insulin. This makes blood sugar management quite challenging.

According to the World Health Organization (WHO), at least 90 % of those with type 2 diabetes are overweight or obese. The longer you have a high body mass index (BMI), the higher your risk of developing type 2 diabetes. Understand that the fat tissues are actively releasing and responding to hormones that increase the risk of one developing metabolic syndrome – including diabetes. This means that, when you lose at least 10-15 pounds, you make a significant difference in your health and blood sugar levels.

If you ask anyone that has tried to lose weight and keep it off sustainably, they will tell you it isn't a joke!

However, this does not mean it is impossible. The truth is, it is possible to lose weight and keep it off. And this is a great benefit to those with diabetes. However, one question most people ask me is, "how do I get started?"

According to experts, the best way to get started is to incorporate a healthy diet into your overall health management regimen – and that is what helped me a great deal.

Here are some steps that worked for me, and hope that they will work for you too;

Step 1 Set small and realistic goals.

Most people fail to realize that losing weight is one thing, but keeping it off is a whole different ballgame. While you want to see, the pounds fall off in a few days of dieting, making drastic changes with your diets and extreme workouts have proven unsustainable.

If you look at the previous chapter on weight loss challenge, you will see that the workouts and changes you make in your diet are not extreme, but they are not also your usual – hence the reason it is a challenge.

The point here is to focus on changes you can sustainably maintain in the long-term.

I will let you in on a secret – you cannot transform your body all at once. That can be a recipe for disaster. The best trick is to set small but realistic goals you can work towards achieving them. You can start by taking a walk around the block at least four times a week instead of doing it every day.

If you do that, these goals will soon become habits, and you can move on to the next objective. This will make you feel a sense of accomplishment even as you progress with your weight loss goals. Remember, setbacks happen to all of us. So, don't let them discourage you from giving up!

Step 2 Get active

One of the most important factors for losing weight is diet. Exercise, on the other hand, is the key to keeping that weight off sustainably. The truth is, when I increased physical activity and a significant reduction in calorie intake, I lost more body fat.

To lose that weight and keep it off, you must aim for at least 150 minutes of moderate workouts a week spread out through the week. Note that fitness does not necessarily mean you must sweat for hours working out. The trick is to find ways to stay active throughout the day. You can choose to walk during lunch breaks at work, park farther away from your destination to add up on those steps, or take the stairs instead of a lift. I work from my basement office. I keep a bottle of water and keep drinking water. Every 30 minutes, I go up one floor to my residence on the ground floor to use it. This way, I can climb up and come down at least 15 times and give me a 5 minutes break from sitting in front of my laptop. All these incremental adjustments to your routine will make a difference in your weight and diabetes condition.

Step 3 Schedule your meals the right way – plus breakfast.

One of the things most people trying to lose weight don't know is that breakfast is key. If you don't take your breakfast, then you risk overeating later in the day. This is something that risks sabotaging your weight loss plans and causing a fluctuation in your blood sugar levels. Taking your breakfast faithfully will help boost your energy to stay active throughout the day.

While the importance of morning meals pertaining to weight loss has been subject to debates, one study published in Advances in Nutrition, September 2014, demonstrated that eating breakfast is linked to weight loss. According to experts, consuming your breakfast – diabetes diet – ensures that your body makes good insulin use throughout the day.

What helped me lose weight was eating a fiber-rich, zero carb diet for breakfast, whey protein, or four boiled eggs with a green salad to help keep your blood sugar levels in check. Ensure that before you buy any foods, you check the labels. Skip cereals and anything else that has added sugars.

Step 4 Cut calories

It is one thing to not consume any carbs in your diet but is quite another to consume too many calories in you. Diet by eating too many fats. Realize that while fats are good for your body, an excess of it can be converted into sugars, raising your glucose levels in the blood.

Therefore, cutting down on your caloric intake goes a long way in helping you achieve weight loss.

I would recommend that you work closely with a registered dietitian or diabetes educator to help you figure out the best diet plan that will suit your goals, tastes, and lifestyle. They will help you determine the right number of calories based on a wide range of factors like age, current weight, body type, gender, and activity levels. This way, you lose weight, keep it off, and manage your blood glucose levels appropriately.

Step 5 Feast on fiber

Now that we have mentioned why it is necessary to cut back on your caloric intake, it is not always easy. This is especially the case when you are hungry soon after you are through with your meals.

The trick is to introduce fiber into your diet because the body will not always be able to break down plant-based carbohydrates. This means that the digestive system will be slow in breaking down food. In effect, the blood sugar levels will be under control.

Realize that foods that are loaded with fiber tend to have low levels of calories. This means that you can eat large quantities of fiber than other foods and still have the same number of calories. Considering fiber takes a long time to get digested, they will keep you fuller for longer.

According to a study published in the Journal of Nutrition, June 2019, people who consume large quantities of fiber have a high likelihood of sticking to a low-calorie diet for longer and lose weight more.

The US Department of Agriculture recommends that women between the ages of 31-50 should consume less than 25 grams of fiber. Men, on the other hand, should consume at least 31 grams of fiber daily.

As you age, your caloric intake and nutrient requirements decline. If you are a woman above 51 years old, your dietary fiber intake should be 22 grams a day while men in the same bracket should consume less than 28 grams daily.

Unfortunately, most people don't even go anywhere near these USDA guidelines.

If you want to lose weight and improve your diabetes situation, the trick is to incorporate fiber-rich foods into your diet. Have legumes, veggies, nuts, and millets in your diet plan.

Step 6 Keep track of your goals and progress.

The other thing I learned in my weight loss journey is the importance of writing down every detail of your journey. This will help you set healthy, realistic, and achievable targets and note the patterns as you progress. This way, you will appreciate small milestones along the way while also taking note of when your diet might have gone off track.

Write down all the foods you eat and the portions per serving. If you are thinking, "oh no, I am not a fan of pen and paper," then try one of the many free apps available online. Weigh yourself at least once in a week to keep track of progress. Include your workout exercises, how you did them, and how you felt about them. I use my fitness pall app to record my diet and exercise every day.

Step 7 Get support

What I learned about my weight loss journey is that I couldn't have done it without my friends, family, and workout buddies. Staying motivated to stick to the plan without losing sight of the end goal – weight loss and improved diabetes – can be tough if you go alone.

When you connect with others, you get the emotional support you need to keep going. Most weight loss programs are usually founded on the concept that support groups/networks play a significant role in staying motivated.

Realize that support comes in a wide range of forms. It could be an online support group, while others can get it from their friends and family. Whatever works well for you, go for it as long as you don't lose sight of your end goal.

Step 8 Avoid overeating using these tricks.

Some of the strategies that will help you avoid overeating or even indulging in foods that will ruin your diet include;

Filling up on low-calorie foods. Simply start with those foods that are lowest in calories and fill a large portion of your plate. The best ones are the non-starchy veggies. This ensures that you will not be so hungry by the time you get to the other foods.

Change your salad dressing system. Rather than pouring dressing on your salads, the trick is to dip into a side dish of dressing before you bite. I was amazed at how much calories I saved and how much less I used. Do the same.

If you feel idle, instead of staying inactive, simply take up a busy-hand hobby. This way, you lower your chances of eating when you are not hungry. Keep yourself occupied with such activities as walking, scrapbooking, knitting, gardening, or crossword puzzles.

Arrive fashionably to parties. When you don't have much time to indulge with the buffet table and calorie-rich appetizers, you are less likely to over-indulge.

That said, losing weight and keeping it off starts with your mindset. If you foster a positive mindset, you make it easy to stick to a healthy diet and regular workout routines, even once you achieve your weight loss goals. The most important thing is that you set SMART goals from the beginning. The healthy habits you initiate for the sake of losing weight will last a lifetime if you keep working at it every step of the journey, and will be the reason you keep that weight off and improve your overall wellbeing. Nowadays, whenever we have any party at home, I just pick up the snacks which work for me best. I don't touch rice, bread, desserts, or any other carbs. I just pick up only proteins. This way, I don't miss anything, and at the same time, I eat right what suits me.

Chapter 8 Intermittent fasting for weight loss

First of all, intermittent fasting is not a diet!

It helps to think of intermittent fasting as a timed-approach to eating. Unlike other dietary plans, you know that restrict caloric intake and the sources thereof; this approach does not specify the kind of food you should eat or avoid. It involves cycling between eating and fasting periods.

Even though intermittent fasting was at the forefront of helping me lose weight, one thing you must realize is that it is not sustainable for everyone. When getting started, most people find it challenging to eat during short intervals every day or even alternating between non-eating and eating days.

In this chapter, we will delve deeper into what intermittent fasting truly means, what it entails, and how best you can use it to achieve your weight loss goals. Popularly, this approach is known to simplify life, lose weight, and boost your overall health and wellbeing while also promoting the quality of life.

One thing you must note is that intermittent fasting is not just another weight loss strategy or hack bodybuilders use to shed off extra fat fast. At its best, this approach is a healthy lifestyle that is informed by our evolution as humans, as well as the study of metabolism. It asks you to be more efficient and protective as opposed to being flowing with the fads of modern times.

Think about it – do you know what happens in your body when you fast?

The truth is, there are many things that happen whenever we fast compared to those that happen during fed states. When it comes to current weight loss trends, intermittent fasting takes center stage. There are tons of celebrities – Stassi Schroeder, Halle Berry, Vanessa Hudgens, and Jenna Jameson – out there who swear by intermittent fasting for weight loss. I am no celebrity, but I have successfully lost weight using intermittent fasting as part of my weight loss strategy.

That said, the benefits of this approach are not limited to weight loss. According to research, this method helps lower the blood cholesterol levels, promotes better sleep, and improves concentration.

If you plan on using intermittent fasting for weight loss, you must understand that it is pretty easy to do it incorrectly. Some people say that they use intermittent fasting but do not see the results in their weight. If done incorrectly, It has the potential of stalling your weight loss. The trick here is to ensure that you nail your eating window to ensure that you reap maximum results in your weight and overall health. In other words, the timing and type of food you eat when you break your fast matters most.

Perhaps you are wondering, "how does it work for weight loss, precisely?"

Understand that intermittent fasting is all about **when** you eat. Depending on the If approach you choose to go with, you can either shorten the fed state or engage in approximately 24-hours of fasting at least once or more times in a week. The most popular approaches include the 16:8, 5:2, 12-hour fast, and others, we will discuss further later in this chapter.

When you restrict your food intake to a shortened time window, what you are doing is lowering your caloric intake, hence promoting weight loss. At the most basic, you must remember that weight loss happens when you consume fewer calories compared to what you expend at the end of the day. You are not only taking in fewer calories but also slowing down the insulin pump, which in turn promotes fat burning.

"So, how long then does it take to start losing weight when you are doing intermittent fasting?" You ask.

That is a very good question!

Unfortunately – or depending on how you look at it - weight is not achieved by a single factor. There are lots of factors that contribute to the length of time it takes to shed off those extra pounds. The rate of weight loss varies from one person to the other based on your starting weight, types of food you eat during the eating window, your intermittent fasting approach, and many more.

If you end up lowering your overall caloric intake immediately and consistently consume fewer calories than you lose, then it is only logical that you lose weight immediately. However, there is a high chance you will not notice immediate weight loss results at least for a couple of weeks. The main reason is that during the beginning of your weight loss journey, most of what you will lose is water weight.

Most experts explain that depending on the number of calories you eat during your intermittent fasts; there is a chance you will experience about 1-2 pounds of weight loss every week. This simply means that it can take upwards of 8-10 weeks before you can notice any significant change in your weight loss.

If you lose more than that, it is a red flag. In short, if you lose a noticeable amount of weight during the initial weeks of intermittent fasting, it is advisable to evaluate your caloric intake to ensure that your nutrition is not jeopardized. As much as you want to lose weight, you must realize that your body's nutrition still comes first.

You may be thinking, "so, I'm doing intermittent fasting but not losing weight. What could be the problem?" Some of the possible mistakes you are making include;

Eating too much during the feeding window.

Remember, weight loss comes down to the number of calories in vs. calories out. If you consume an equal number of calories or more during your fed state compared to what you started with during intermittent fasting, the chances are that you will not lose any weight. Let's face it - if you pack all the calories you normally consume during your eating window, the truth is that you are not changing your diet one bit.

To fix this, try using a calorie-counting app. Even though I don't normally recommend the use of apps in counting your calories, it goes a long way in helping you keep track of your caloric intake – at least for a couple of days. The app will normally tell you the approximate number of calories you need to start losing weight.

Even though these estimations are not usually accurate, they can help point you in the right direction. They can reveal meals or foods that are high in caloric content than you initially thought so that you can adjust accordingly.

Not consuming adequate calories during non-fasting days.

You are thinking, "isn't that the whole point of losing weight?"

While you want to lose weight, it helps to ensure that you consume an adequate number of calories when you are not fasting. The truth is, your body may conserve the energy you consume instead of burning it.

To fix this, ensure that you create a meal plan for non-fasting days. Ensure that the meal plan includes a balanced diet consisting of at least 300-500 calories per meal. This way, your body will not have to resort to guesswork. Therefore, don't skimp calories for yourself!

Loading up on less-nutritious foods

Even though the main focus on intermittent fasting is **when** you eat instead of **what** you eat, it doesn't mean that you can pump your body with whatever you wish to have during your eating period. Remember, you are still on a weight loss journey, and you don't get to eat whatever you want and expect to have a successful weight loss journey. If your diet is loaded with calorie-dense foods, you can forget about losing weight.

To achieve your weight loss goals, it is best if you focus on consuming nutrient-dense foods. When you pump your body with foods that are rich in fiber carbs, lean proteins, and healthy fats, you will naturally be filled up, and your overall caloric-intake will decline.

No cheat days!

Not fasting long enough.

If you decide on a specific time-restricted feeding method and you shorten your eating window by saying an hour per day, there is a high likelihood you will not see much – if any weight loss at all. To lose weight, you must be willing to change enough from your usual eating routine.

Research shows that most women draw success from a 10-hour eating window, which means a 14-hour fasting state. The best thing is to try with a longer eating window and then work your way down, especially if your eating window is normally longer than this.

Skipping meals during your eating window

One mistake most people make is thinking that by skipping meals, they will lose lots of weight. One thing you must note is that skipping meals and not consuming enough when you are supposed to eat will only push you to extreme hunger, especially during fasting periods. This means that when you are supposed to be fasting, your extreme hunger will push you to break your fasts. Restricting yourself excessively during the eating windows risk overeating and bingeing during your next eating window, causing a high caloric intake than is needed.

The best trick here is to ensure that you are eating to your fill during eating windows. Don't get me wrong – I am not saying that you should overstuff yourself with food during eating windows. With a proper meal plan in place, you will ensure that you don't skip meals whenever you are busy or thrown off schedule and that when you eat, you get the required portion – nothing less, nothing more – just enough!

Choosing the wrong type of fasting plan

There are various types of intermittent fasting plans. All these plans are not the same, and not all of them will fit your lifestyle or boost your metabolic rate. Let us consider an instance where you are training for an endurance challenge. In that case, you will not go for a plan that prevents you from eating in the morning when you need fuel for your workout. If you do it, then you risk falling off the wagon in the process, harm your body and performance too.

The best trick here is to consider choosing an intermittent fasting plan that best suits your lifestyle. You want a plan you can maintain for the long haul. For me, it was easy to fast during the night for 12 hours. I take my dinner at 9 pm and eat breakfast the next day after 9 am only. I start with one tablespoon of cold press coconut oil and green tea, followed by a salad. I also fast every Monday from lunch to lunch the next day. That means I will have a good breakfast and lunch on Monday and have the next very lite meal as lunch, starting with a spoon of cold-pressed coconut oil.

Also, consult with your dietitian to ensure that the decision you make is based on a proper assessment of your lifestyle and dietary requirements.

Insufficient enough sleep

Very few studies have focused on assessing the direct correlation between sleep and weight loss when one is on an intermittent fasting plan. However, several research studies have demonstrated a connection between sleep and positive weight loss results.

The best trick here is to try to get at least 7 – 9 hours of sleep per night. Yes, this might be tough at first, but ensure that you do your best. Your weight loss goals and overall wellbeing depend on it!

Working out too much

I don't know about you, but I have seen many people start a new eating plan at the same time they start a workout plan. You may not be on a new exercise plan, but the chances are that you have increased the intensity of your workouts just the same time you are getting started on a new diet plan.

What you don't know is that over-exercising while lowering your food intake has a significant impact on your energy levels. In other words, your energy levels go down, and your hunger pangs skyrocket. This sets you at risk of overeating, hence consuming more calories during your eating windows.

The best way to fix this is by practicing full-day or full-night fasts while keeping your exercises light on fasting days. Generally, it is advisable to ensure that your workout regimen is challenging while still doable and enjoyable when you are fasting. If you notice that you are hungry on workout days, it simply indicates that you are pushing yourself too much.

Lack of proper hydration

If you don't keep yourself properly hydrated, especially during fasting days, the chances are that you will be dehydrated. You miss out on the benefits that water has to offer, like quelling hunger.

Ensure that you drink up. The good thing with intermittent fasting is that you can get a little fancy with your water. For instance, you can choose to have iced tea, coffee with stevia, hot tea, black coffee, and much more.

Deviating from the plan, you are instructed to follow.

It is true that following an intermittent fasting plan down to the last detail can be challenging for most people. There are people who choose to go for long durations before eating anything at all. If you keep cheating on your plan every other week or cutting corners here and there, there is a high likelihood it will not yield the weight loss results you are hoping for. That means you might want to reconsider if intermittent fasting really suits your lifestyle or not/

If not, it is best to go for an intermittent fasting plan that suits your lifestyle better and one you can stick to for longer durations.

Not planning ahead

One of the most important aspects of any type of health intervention is proper planning ahead. If you don't have a plan, then it is easy to get swayed into settling for just about anything – including unhealthy eating habits.

Today, choose to plan all your meals and snacks ahead of time. When you have a plan of what to prepare, when, and how to do it, you make it easy to stick to your health plan and ultimately achieve your weight loss goals. If you don't have a plan, the chances are that you will settle for a restaurant menu to decide what to eat from time to time – or maybe all the time!

Feelings of guilt for breaking the fast.

You must note that intermittent fasting is an approach that calls for practice and patience. Several people who try intermittent fasting – regardless of the method they choose – end up breaking the fast before the schedule at some point in their fast. If you are really serious about sticking to intermittent fasting for weight loss, you must learn not to feel guilty, angry, or ashamed when you break the fast. Accept that you are human and get back up on your regular program as soon as you can.

Give yourself a little grace and move on. Constantly remind yourself that intermittent fasting takes a number of trial and errors, and this is one of them. Realize that errors in intermittent fasting are inevitable, and there will be times when you won't be able to avoid them even if you try hard.

Forgive yourself and move on!

Don't allow it cause you to lose sight of the end goal – weight loss and improved wellbeing!

Intermittent fasting methods

The 16/8 method

This is a fasting method that involves an everyday fast for at least 16 hours and then restricting your daily eating window to 8 hours. During the eating window, you can at least fit in 2 or more meals; a method referred to as the Leangains protocol. This method was popularized by Martin Berkhan, a fitness expert.

The thing with this method of fasting is that it can be as simple as skipping dinner and not eating until the following day. For instance, if you have your last meal at 6 pm, you don't eat anything until 2 pm the following day, which technically is 16 hours.

That said, experts recommend that women fast for only 14 hours because they do better with shorter fasts. If you like having your breakfast – which is highly recommended – this method may be a little challenging to get used to at first. However, for those who skip breakfast, they do this instinctively. You may also opt to have water, coffee, or a calorie-free beverage during the fast to lower the feelings of hunger.

One thing you must bear in mind is that you are fasting to lose weight. In that case, it is important that you eat healthy foods during your eating window. If you eat junk foods or excessive calories, there is no way you will achieve your weight loss goals.

The 5:2 diet

This method involves eating for five days a week and then restricting calories to only 500-600 calories for the other remaining two days. This diet is also referred to as the fast diet. 5:2 diet is a method that was popularized by Michael Mosley, a British Journalist.

During your fasting days, you are required to eat 500 calories for women and 600 calories if you are a man.

For instance, you may choose to eat normally for five days a week except Thursday and Monday. For these fasting days, you can eat small meals of 250 calories – for women – or 300 calories – for men.

That said, there are no studies that have tested the 5:2 diet method itself. However, there are plenty of studies that have demonstrated the importance of using intermittent fasting for weight loss – and that is what matters most.

Eat-stop-eat

This is a method that involves fasting for 24 hours once or twice a week. It is a fasting method that was popularized by Brad Pilon, a fitness expert. This is method has been very popular over the past few years. Here, you fast from dinner one day to dinner the following day, which adds up to 24 hours.

For instance, if you finish your dinner at say 8 pm on Monday, you don't eat anything thereafter until 8 pm dinner the following day. In other words, once you decide to fast, you have to stop eating until 24 hours lapses since your last meal. You can also do this from breakfast to breakfast or lunch to lunch because the end result is the same.

During the fast, you can have water, coffee, or other calorie-free beverages. However, solid foods are not allowed here. To achieve weight loss, you must ensure that your eating is normal during the eating window. In short, eat the same quantity of the food as though you had not been fasting in the first place.

There is one potential downside to this fasting method – it can be really difficult for many people to pull off a 24 hour fast. However, you don't necessarily have to go all-in at once. You can start with 14-15 hours and then slowly work your way up to 24 hours.

You can do it!

Alternate-day fasting

This is a method that involves fasting every other day. There is a wide range of versions of this method. There are some that allow approximately 500 calories during the fasting days. According to research, many of the test tube studies have demonstrated the health benefits of using this version of intermittent fasting.

While a full fast every day is extreme, this is something that is not recommended for beginners. The thing with this method is that you can go to bed hungry several days a week, making it unpleasant and unsustainable in the long term.

The warrior diet

This is a method that was popularized by Ori Hofmekler, a fitness expert, and was one of the most popular diets to be included as a form of intermittent fasting. Here, you are supposed to eat small quantities of veggies and raw fruits during the day and then one large meal at night.

In other words, you can fast all day and then feast at night – within a four-hour eating window. The food choices, in this case, are quite similar to those eaten on a paleo diet, in short, whole, unprocessed foods.

Spontaneous meal skipping

With spontaneous meal skipping, you don't necessarily need a structured fasting plan to enjoy all the benefits of an intermittent fast. The most common option here is that you skip meals from time to time. For instance, when you don't feel hungry or are too busy to cook or can't find time to go eat.

One misconception people have is that you need to eat every couple of hours, or else you will hit a starvation mode or start losing your muscles. The truth is, your body is well-equipped to go long hours without food, let alone just a meal or two skipped once in a while.

Therefore, if you don't really feel hungry, simply skip that meal – preferably lunch or dinner. Remember, breakfast is the most important meal of the day, and it is highly recommended that you don't skip it at all. Additionally, if you are traveling and can't find anything to eat, simply use that opportunity for a short fast.

When you skip one or two meals when you feel like doing, it is simply referred to as spontaneous intermittent fasting. The most important thing is that you eat healthy foods when you actually want to eat – during meal times.

Remember, intermittent fasting is one of the best weight loss tools that has worked for me and will work for you too. While there are people who believe that it is not beneficial to women as it is for men, what I know is that it is not recommended for people with eating disorders. If you decide to try any of the above intermittent fasting methods, bear in mind that diet quality is a game-changer. You cannot binge on junk foods during your eating window and expect that you will lose weight and improve your overall wellbeing.

Stages of Intermittent fasting

When in a well-fed state, your body cells are active in a growth model. In most cases, insulin signals the mTOR pathways that tell the cells to grow, divide, and make proteins. In short, the cells in the body are active. This mTOR loves a plentiful supply of nutrients – carbs and proteins. When active, mTOR signals the cells not to bother with self-eating – otherwise referred to as autophagy. This is a recycling and cleanup process that helps the body get rid of damaged and misfolded proteins.

Here, the well-fed cells are not really worried about efficiency because they are busy growing and dividing.

The most important thing to note here is that well-fed cells are highly acetylated, which means that proteins responsible for wrapping DNA up nicely into the core of the cell – histones – are adorned with lysine and acetyl groups on them.

You are wondering, "what on earth are all these things you are talking about?"

Don't worry – my point here is that well-fed cells comprise many genes, including those responsible for proliferation and cellular survival. The main reason is that acetylation tends to package proteins loosely in the cells, which means that your DNA can easily be read for protein production.

During fasting, your cells turn on the genes responsible for proliferation and cellular growth and turn off other genes – like those responsible for fat metabolism, damage repair, and stress resistance. You must understand that when you are fasting, all fats are turned into ketones that reactivate these genes and contribute to stress resistance and reduced inflammations in the brain.

When you are starving, things are different. The body
reacts to what it perceives from the surroundings – low
availability of food. It does so by changing the expression
of certain genes important for protection against stress.
The system in action here is the AMPK signaling pathway,
which serves as a brake pedal to mTOR's gas pedal. It
signals the cells to go into a self-protective mode, hence
activating the autophagy and breakdown of fat. It also
inhibits mTOR and causes the levels of NAD+ to rise
following the fact that you lack dietary sugars and proteins
required for its conversion through the Krebs cycle.

The ketones released during fasting are also used as a
deacetylase inhibitor, which turns on genes related to
damage repair and antioxidant processes.

See? There is really a lot happening when your body is not
taking calories in the diet. However, the most important
question you might ask is, when exactly do these things
take place? Here are a series of stages that will help you
visualize that better;

Stage 1 Ketosis

After 12 hours of intermittent fasting, your body
automatically enters a state of ketosis. Here, the body
breaks down body fat for use as an energy source. Some of
these fats are used by life for the production of ketone

bodies, which fuels the brain, heart, and skeletal muscle when glucose is absent.

The ketone bodies generated by the liver during fasting state replaces the glucose fuel for the brain and other body organs. The use of ketones by the brain is part of the reason fasting is known to promote mental clarity while promoting a positive mood. Ketones have been shown to produce less inflammatory products during metabolism compared to glucose, and hence kickstart the brain's growth factor BNDF. They also lower cellular damage and cell death in the neurons while also lowering the rate of inflammation.

Stage 2 Fat-burning mode

After about 18 hours of fasting, the body switches into a fat-burning mode, which promotes significant ketones. At this point, blood ketone levels are detected to be above the baseline (0.05 to 0.1 mM). When you fast, you simply restrict the carb diet, and the concentration of ketones rises to 5-7 mM.

As the levels of ketones in the blood rises, they signal the body to ramp up stress-busting pathways that repair damaged DNA and lowers inflammations.

Stage 3 Autophagy

Within 24 hours of fasting, the body cells start recycling old components and break down proteins that have been misfolded. These proteins are often linked to Alzheimer's and other diseases.

One thing you must note about autophagy is that it plays a key role in cellular and tissue rejuvenation. When the cells fail to initiate autophagy, the body starts suffering from severe conditions like neurodegenerative diseases.

The thing with intermittent fasting is that it activates the AMPK signaling pathway that inhibits mTOR activity, hence activating autophagy. On the other hand, when you deplete glucose stores, the insulin levels in the blood begin to drop.

According to a study conducted in mice deprived of food, the rate of autophagy increased after 24 hours, and the effect in the liver and brain cells was magnified after 48 hours. In humans, autophagy is more pronounced in neutrophils after 24 hours of fasting. When you work out and restrict the intake of calories during fasting, the rate of autophagy also increases in the body tissues.

Stage 4 Growth hormone secretion

After 48 hours of fasting – without calories in the body –
the levels of growth hormones increase at least five times
higher than normal. The main reason for this is that the
ketone bodies produced during fasting trigger secretion of
these growth hormones. For instance, the secretion of
ghrelin – the hunger hormone – promotes the growth
hormone secretion, which helps in the preservation of lean
muscle mass while also lowering the accumulation of fat
tissues. It also promotes mammalian longevity, cardio
health, and wound healing.

Stage 5 Increased insulin sensitivity

After 54 hours of fasting, the insulin levels by now have
dropped to its lowest levels. At this point, the body is
quickly becoming more insulin sensitive. Lowering insulin
levels is accompanied by a wide range of health benefits –
both short- and long-term.

One of them is that low levels of insulin put brakes on
insulin and mTOR signaling pathways, hence activating
autophagy. Additionally, low levels of insulin lower
inflammations and protects you against chronic diseases of
aging like cancer.

After 72 hours of fasting, the body starts breaking down old immune cells and starts generating new ones.

Stage 6 Refeeding

This is perhaps the last most important stage of intermittent fasting. When you break your fast, the key to starting right is to eat a nutritious and balanced meal to improve the functioning of your body cells and tissues after undergoing a cleanup process during fasting.

When you eat, the carbs you take in stimulate the release of the incretin hormone glucagon-like peptide one from the endocrine cells of the gut. This hormone enhances the clearance of glucose from the blood by stimulating the secretion of insulin from the pancreas. This results in increased insulin sensitivity of the cells. The thing with this hormone is that it crosses the blood-brain barrier, acts directly on the neurons, and promotes cognition, synaptic plasticity, and cellular stress resistance.

That said, this is not a recommendation to break your fast with loads of carbs and sugars. If you do, it can result in dangerous spikes in blood sugar levels. The best way to break your fast is to eat a healthy and well-balanced meal packed with plant fats, veggies, fibers, whole

grains/legumes, and healthy proteins. The trick is to learn
what works best for you – and don't tell me processed
carbs and sugars.

So, try out one of the different intermittent fasting
methods we have discussed and above and watch how that
impacts your weight loss and overall wellbeing.

Chapter 9 Burning fat using High-Intensity interval training (HIIT)

Perhaps you are thinking, *"to cardio or not to cardio?"*

Well, unless you love running on a treadmill for hours or joins marathons willingly just to have fun, there is a chance that you will have a hard time finding workouts that push your cardio fitness to its fullest without necessary taking a whole day to complete.

The good news is that you don't have to grind out hours of your day trying to burn fats. The main reason is that you have HIIT – High-intensity interval training – that will help you achieve your cardio fitness in just a short time. HIIT is often referred to as an all-out workout that requires exhaustive physical effort just for a short duration. In other instances, it is active recovery.

According to research, aerobic HIIT has been shown to increase VO2max compared to other aerobic training done continuously in spite of the fact that HIIT takes a short time to complete. Moreover, a study published in the Journal of Strength and conditioning reported that engaging in HIIT rowing for a month straight has the ability to burn more body fats compared to traditional rowing.

One thing you must remember is that when done well, HIIT can be a saving cardio grace. It has the potential of delivering a lot of the results you are looking for – elevated heart rate, fat burning, improved lung capacity, and pushing you to sweat. You can achieve all these and more in just a fraction of time, hence considered a very useful workout for people who prefer not to spend all day in the gym.

That said, you must be willing to utilize HIIT correctly and ensure that your intensity is high for you to enjoy all these benefits. What I love most about this workout is that it did not only help me shed extra pounds in a short time but also the fact that it is far from boring. Its work-to-rest ratios make this workout time efficient, especially when it comes to burning calories. Using HIIT, you can build an entire workout plan or apply just a couple of sets to the super-charged finisher.

What makes this workout unique is the high intensity involved. Here, you are going as hard as you can for a short duration before you take time out to rest and recover before you go hard again. Remember, this is the work-to-rest ration workout, and there are a number of rations you can consider depending on what you wish to achieve;

1:2 or 1:1 work-to-rest rations for at least 30 seconds work and 30 seconds rest is acceptable if you wish to improve your aerobic fitness. On the other hand, if you wish to train anaerobically – mostly sport-specific training for explosiveness and power – you can take longer rest intervals for maximal effort. This often takes a 1:5 ratio, which is 15 seconds of work and 75 seconds work.

The key to HIIT

The key here is the intensity. One thing that must bear in mind is that you cannot coast through your work durations when doing HIIT. The truth is, HIIT protocols are designed in such a way to offer you a chance to go as hard as you possibly can – and you need to leverage that chance.

In other words, work hard. Don't get me wrong – I am not saying that you should go 100% with your intensity. If you are a beginner, it is advisable that you don't go all out at once. You can take 15 seconds to 30-second intervals performed at nearly 100%, ensuring that the maximum effort you give is around 80% and then a couple of minutes – preferably 5 minutes – of low-intensity workouts. This, according to studies, has been shown to play a significant role in weight loss among the sedentary population.

If you choose to work out in a group fitness setting, the best thing is to alternate between interval training and HIIT. That said, you must remember that true HIIT calls for intense and explosive work periods. However, basic interval training does not involve high-intensity aspects of the workouts with longer rest periods and shorter work periods.

Primary benefits of HIIT

Fat loss

According to a review of over 13 different studies on over 400 obese adults, HIIT and traditional moderate-intensity workouts have been shown to play a significant role in the reduction of waist circumference and weight loss.

HIIT has been shown to serve as a natural booster of the human growth hormone, which is important for optimal strength, health, and vigor. It also has been shown to improve sensitivity to insulin, increased muscle growth, and fat loss.

If you have been on a diet before, then you know that it is nearly impossible not to lose muscle mass along with fat when you are cutting down on calories. That said, studies have demonstrates that 24 hours of HIIT workouts lead to 450% more production of HGH, which encourages the body to build and preserve lean muscle mass while ensuring that it rids the body of excess fat.

Increased efficiency

The thing I love about HIIT is that it offers a similar psychological outcome as long duration cardio in just about a fraction of the time. It taxes both your aerobic and anaerobic fitness as opposed to traditional cardio exercises that only focus on aerobic fitness.

Aerobic fitness increases your oxygen needs whole the anaerobic exercises focus on building your muscles. Both these exercises work together to boost your endurance and ensure that you get stronger simultaneously.

Research studies demonstrate that performing HIIT exercises at least three times a week for as little as 27 minutes offers the same aerobic and anaerobic improvements, just like steady-state cardio workouts performed five times a week for an hour. This way, you can complete your workouts in less time and have more time to go about your everyday life.

Improved stamina

Do you push your body into the anaerobic zone? Most people are not used to pushing themselves hard enough to a point where they can't breathe, and their heart rates feel like the heart is about to jump out of their chests.

One thing you need to realize is that when you push yourself to work out this hard, you are helping your heart work better. Your heart becomes happier – so to speak!

According to a research study conducted in 2006, research participants who worked out for eight weeks had the ability to bicycle twice as much as they could before the study. What is interesting is that they maintained the same pace. The truth is, working out taxes your aerobic and anaerobic systems, hence ensuring that you achieve optimal cardio benefits.

Versatility

Jumping rope, running, and biking work well for HIIT training. However, what you must remember is that you don't need any special equipment to engage in high-intensity workouts. All you need sometimes are fast feet, high knees, and anything plyometric such as jumping lunges. The whole point is to get your heart rate up and fast.

The truth is, using equipment in most cases contributes to a less effective workout. The focus here is to push your heart to its optimal limit, not just one muscle group at a time.

Break mental barriers

When you push your body and brain outside its comfort zones, you are opening yourself to increased mental resiliency. It will allow you to challenge yourself not just during exercise but also in your everyday life increasingly.

By persevering during tough high-intensity exercises, you gain more confidence to face tough challenges in real life – and that means both physical and mental challenges. With this, you will constantly hear your inner voice telling you, "I can do this," and you know what? – Your inner voice couldn't be more accurate!

Increased metabolic rate for hours

According to research, HIIT is said to increase metabolism for several hours after a workout. This is higher compared to the impact of weight training and jogging on metabolic rate – otherwise known as the excess post-exercise oxygen consumption (EPOC).

When EPOC is ignited, the rate of metabolism is increased for at least 48 hours. Considering HIIT training plays a role in building muscle mass because of the muscle cells burning more calories than fat cells, and increased metabolism is achieved. Additionally, research demonstrates that engaging in anaerobic workouts helps boost resting energy consumption.

Scientifically, anaerobic workouts are known to increase the basal metabolic rate – otherwise referred to as the rate of energy the body uses during rest (measured in kJ/hour/kg body mass). Therefore, each time you have a chance to boost your metabolic rate, don't think twice – just do it! It will not only help you lose weight but will also help keep your body healthy both inside and outside.

Overall health

One thing you must note is that HIIT is not just another tool used to lean out. The truth is that it can improve your overall health and wellbeing. According to 50 different studies, HIIT has been shown to lower blood sugar levels. It also has a significant role in lowering the resting heart rate and blood pressure, especially among overweight and obese individuals.

Indeed, with effective HIIT training, you can torch calories, build lean muscle, shed off extra pounds, improve your health, push your limits, and boost your efficiency.

Although these benefits are plentiful, there are still many myths around this type of workout that risk getting in the way of your performance. Let us find out truths to some of the common misconceptions so that you can perform your HIIT perfectly;

Longer is better

Well, this is false.

One thing most people fail to realize is that they do not need more than 30 minutes for a workout to be effective. The idea of HIIT is to ensure that you go all out. Instead of jogging, you sprint. When the duration of your high-intensity exercises approaches half-hour, the truth is that your intensity greatly goes down. Therefore, the next time you plan your HIIT workout session, break down your workouts like this;

Work: 8 min

Rest: 2 min

Work: 7 min

Rest: 2 min

Work: 6 min

Total time: 25 minutes

What if running outdoors is your cup of tea? In that case, you can replace 2.5km of jogging with at least five 500-meter sprints to ensure that you reap all the benefits HIIT has to offer.

All workouts are well-suited for HIIT.

If I have learned anything from HIIT training, it is that not all exercises should be used here. If you truly want to achieve high-intensity, it is advisable to go for full body movements that will tax your cardio system and boost your endurance strength.

For instance, dumbbell snatches, burpees, kettlebell clean and swings, and presses work best on hill sprints.

However, single-joint workouts like triceps extensions and bicep curls are not great at offering full-body conditioning. The guiding principle I use is, if I can talk during a high-intensity interval, then that is not a HIIT exercise.

HIIT alone will shed weight

One of the greatest benefits of HIIT is that it triggers excess post-exercise oxygen consumption – also referred to as afterburn. This plays an important role in boosting the body's rate of metabolism at least for over 48 hours after a high-intensity workout.

However, it does not mean that it is a license to eat all kinds of foods you desire.

Each time you indulge in a cheat meal after training, you can forget about seeing the results you want. Quit using HIIT as a way to rationalize your poor eating habits. The best move is for you to clean up your diet. This way, you get a burst of new energy for your exercises while still enjoy all the results you desire.

HIIT training bulks you up

Just as we mentioned, HIIT will help you burn fat and maintain lean muscles. It will also boost your cardio endurance while ensuring that your work capacity grows. You may be wondering, "but what is work capacity anyway?"

This is simply the ability of the body to work at varying intensities and durations. Remember, muscular hypertrophy can be achieved through bodybuilding training. Therefore, you should not be afraid to clean, swing, or press a heavy kettlebell or even snatch a massive dumbbell. These compound movements will help your entire body by taxing your cardio system, boost your metabolism, and leave you breathless.

You must have fancy equipment to perform HIIT.

The truth is, you don't need fancy equipment to exercise HIIT training. If you don't have dumbbells, you can focus more on getting your heart rate up and keeping it there. These chipper workouts will help you achieve that without any equipment.

The chipper workouts are composed of 60 sit-ups, 50 jump squats, 40 pushups, 30 split jumps, 20 triceps dips, and ten burpees. The best trick is to perform each of these workouts with at least 30 seconds of rest in between. Ensure that you give it your 100% effort and repeat them every day with the aim of completing them faster than the last each time. You can do this by lowering the rest time in between exercises and work faster times.

Chapter 10 Consistency: The key to successful weight loss

The end goal here is to lose weight and get your health and wellbeing back on track, right?

But first, let's forget about all the dangers that excess body fat possess on your health and overall wellbeing. While it is great to lose excess body fat, you must remind yourself that you are a simpler soul with kinder dreams.

We all want to look great or prettier before we start aging. You don't want to live your youthful years with a tired look and a body that does not fit in your beautiful outfits. You want a body that, even when it ages, it still radiates vitality and power.

In short, we all want to live a fuller life – proud and fierce.

Weight loss is all about consistency. There is no space for hating your body or sucking over a lack of self-esteem. You no longer want to feel uncomfortable, lack certainty, and live depressed.

But what is the problem?

The one thing no one ever tells you is you must have consistency. Research shows that over 95% of those who lose weight regain it – all and more! Their bodies fight hard, but they still end up regaining the weight after they had successfully lost it all. In other words, only a small 5% are able to maintain their weight loss goals in the long-term.

These are such unsettling statistics, but the question you must ask yourself is, why work so hard to lose weight only to regain it all back? Why does the lost weight creep back in?

If you pay attention to most weight loss success stories, people are always busy telling half-truths about weight loss. But the one they never manage to tell you is that your consistency is key to losing weight and keeping it off even in the long-term. In every successful weight loss story, there are three keys that are evident;

- Psychological influence to focus your attention on the weight loss you want
- Revitalizing diet habits critical to weight loss
- Workout mastery

These three keys are what make weight watchers unstoppable, but the problem is, how do you lose those extra pounds consistently?

Psychological influence to focus your attention on the weight loss you want

Some of the psychological factors that hold back people from losing weight are the fact that they fail to revisit why they want that extra weight off. People scroll through Google's random pages on how to lose weight and use that as the only source of knowledge.

Don't get me wrong- I am not saying that Google has no good information on weight loss because it is actually a powerful source of credible information. However, what people lack is the insider view of what is working and what is not—in other words, finding real people who actually have lost weight and maintained it for over three years— finding their real experiences, strategies, challenges, and victories that accompanied their weight loss journey. This way, you can gain a deeper insight into why it is really hard to lose weight and keep it off.

Consistency comes from reading scholarly weight loss research studies that have been performed on real people. The most important thing is that you feed your mind with credible life-changing information that will help you embark on a guilty-free weight loss strategy that actually works. With this, you get a chance to discover different forms of energy balance, which will set you apart from all else.

You may be thinking, "I can't even clock enough sleep at night. How can I focus on shedding off extra pounds and keeping it off?"

While it is challenging to stick to good sleep schedules every single day of your life with all the multiple distractions you encounter, if you keep coming up with excuses not to get enough sleep, you need to stop and ask yourself how badly you want to lose weight and get back in shape.

The truth is, getting enough sleep at night is one of the best strategies of losing weight. It keeps the appetite hormones in proper check. If you are sleep-deprived, then you cause an imbalance on these appetite hormones, hence increasing your food cravings, which quickly spin out of control.

Additionally, low quality sleep causes an increase in the release of cortisol, which directs the body to store up fats to help fuel your waking times. In short, sleep deprivation undermines dietary attempts to lose weight.

Today, aim for at least 7-9 hours of sleep per day.

Now, how do you monitor your progress in weight loss? Yes, you stick to your weight loss program, have healthy eating habits, and weigh yourself regularly because you expect tangible outcomes, but how do you keep track of your progress?

One thing you must note is that a weight loss calculator will help you paint a clearer and vivid picture of where you are and how far you are from where you want to be. When you keep a record of your progress, you can easily pinpoint what is not working out for you. This will give you a clear view of the strengths of your approach. Keep track of what you eat every day, what you do, and when, feelings, and moods associated with every moment.

Irrespective of what you wish to achieve, you must set realistic goals. The last thing you want is to feel like you are adrift in the world, working hard, and not seeing the fruits of your labor. The best thing is to take time to examine your weight loss goals and ensure that they are realistic. Realistic simply means that the goals you have set are not only doable but also sustainable with regard to your family, friends, and career. Once six months elapse since you started your weight loss journey, reevaluate your goals to ensure that you are on track. If not, ensure that you adjust where necessary.

Remember, you cannot get it all by yourself. Therefore, don't forget to surround yourself with people who will have your back and cheer you on until you get where you want to be. Don't get me wrong – I am not saying that it is wrong to go at it alone. Support does not just come from others. It can be derived from your day, household, and work environment.

This simply means that you don't bring junk foods into the house if it triggers you to backslide. It can also mean planning out your snack and travel times appropriately, not to allow yourself to go long without meals that you get too hungry. It is deciding to take care of yourself every minute of the day – round the clock.

If there are habits that are not working, now is the time to ditch them. Remember the old adage, "old habits die hard?" there are times on your weight loss journey when you will feel like quitting and going back to your junk, old diet, and sleeping late. However, you must remind yourself that this is not going to help you lose weight successfully.

The truth is that old habits tend to slow down, and there is no way you can go back to doing things the old way. When you take slow but sure steps towards weight loss, you will pay attention to every habit you have that undermines the consistency of your weight loss. This way, you can easily turn them around by taking manageable steps you can handle without feeling like you are suffocating.

For instance, I started by changing the snacks I carry in my bag – cookies and potato chips – to healthy keto snacks. Each night, instead of loading up on what used to be my favorite calorie-free drink, I replaced it with water with a dash of lime. Eventually, I started moving in the right direction, one step at a time. Don't allow those unhealthy snacks in your pantry if you know you cannot control yourself from indulging.

Just don't!

Keep off any gimmicks. While this sounds easy at first, realize that people succumb to pitfalls because so many weight loss fads out there tend to sabotage minds. The truth is, gimmicks are usually the reason weight loss is challenging. You will hear people talk of losing 20 pounds in less than a week, weight loss wonder pills, and a ton of other fads flooding the internet.

You must ask yourself whether these things are even real, and if it is real, why are people not losing weight?

The truth is, there are many things people are not telling you. All you get online are half-truths and quick fixes that don't deliver the results they promised to. They are just out there to waste your time and money while they go on to earn from your clicks.

When I chose to start losing weight, I shut out all the gimmicks so that I could consistently focus on my weight loss strategies for permanent weight loss.

You are wondering, "why are people not getting their weight off despite trying all the tips?"

If you are on a healthy diet, working out and monitoring your caloric intake, and still the scale does not reflect your efforts, the problem might really be on your strategy but instead on your hormones. There are two hormones that are known to undermine weight loss efforts – thyroid hormone deficiency – causing hypothyroidism – and cortisol – the stress hormone.

Let's see how each of these hormones affects weight loss;

Thyroid hormone

The role of this hormone is to regulate metabolism. When this hormone is deficient in the body, that is when you experience a decline in metabolism. This results in weight gain. The good thing is that this does not exceed 15 pounds. The best thing is to have your physician take a blood test to measure the concentration of your thyroid-stimulating hormone. That said, you can prevent this deficiency from happening by loading up on enough iodine from shellfish, fish, iodized salts, and sea veggies.

Cortisol

While this can be a little intimidating, the truth is that we all go through moments of stress. The stresses in our lives trigger the release of cortisol, which increases the levels of sugar in the body for use by the muscles. When these sugars are underutilized, they are converted into fats, hence limiting weight loss progress.

Finally, weight loss requires that you stay mindful. This is a practice that calls for your focus on the present moments. Every minute of your life, bring your thoughts and feelings to your present. This way, you will not only monitor your eating habits but also live healthy and happy as you lose weight.

When you are mindful, you become aware of your physical sensations of hunger, monitor stress, and promote healthy eating habits – all of which are at the core of weight loss.

Consistently revitalizing diet habits critical to weight loss.

Often, I hear people say that they are confused between dieting and working out. Their confusion is that they can't tell which one of the two determines the depth of weight loss.

One thing you must note is that working out or exercising is supplemental to weight loss. However, dieting is a consistent predictor of weight loss. When you lose weight, you are creating a caloric deficit in the body. The more you focus on creating that sustainable deficit, the more successful you are at losing weight.

Don't get me wrong – I am not saying that an extreme diet is a way to go as far as weight loss. Research shows that extreme diets have a fatal effect on one's health by depriving you of major nutrients. Even though you may experience weight loss on an extreme diet, you risk gaining back all the lost weight considering you cannot live on such a diet for life.

My advice would be to think of food as a budget and then be frugal with your strategy. Spend more calories on foods that work well for your body and then set aside a little extra for your carvings. The most important thing you must note about dieting is that when you start, you will lose weight on a weekly basis, and then it slows down gradually as you progress. In the end, your body becomes fully adjusted to your caloric intake, and weight loss stops. At this point, it is advisable to seek exercises to help push you forward towards a lower caloric intake.

I hear some people saying that counting calories do not work, claiming that all calories are not the same. If you do this, then you are not going to lose weight, and you wonder why. Imagine taking 500 calories of garbage. In the next half-hour, you will be hungry and risk overeating. But think about it, if you eat 500 calories of veggies and lean chicken or fish, you will be fully stuffed.

The point here is, if you don't count your calories, you will not be able to keep track of what you load your body with. The whole point of counting your calories is to gain a deeper understanding of what you eat.

Simply start by splitting your daily portions several times and then spread them throughout the day. Ensure that you have your breakfast every day and do not skip any meals. If you do, then you will starve later, and that hunger will risk you overeating.

What worked well for me was keeping my lunches at 400 calories and below. In that case, it is best to go with something that is filling like Spinach or Mixed Vegetables soup. Then have a 150-calorie snack – like a 100 grams of cottage cheese, or one scoo[of whey protein shake – to take you through the rest of the afternoon. Then make your dinner to be around 1000 calories and under. Also, have a 150-calorie snack to take you through the rest of the evening.

To achieve sustainable weight loss, it is important that you make it a habit to load up on weight loss-friendly diets. Bring on fibers and shun processed sugary foods, refined carbs, cookies, and white bread. Pack your plate with fiber-filled fruits, whole grains, and veggies, which filling and satisfying for longer.

That said, don't say that because this is a healthy food, you can have a plate full or several plates for that matter. The more you consume, the more calories you are packing onto your body. I might have said this before, eat from small-sized plates to give you an illusion that you have taken a bigger portion already. This way, your subconscious mind will tell you that you have already taken a big portion, and that is enough.

Additionally, bring everyone in your household on board with your weight loss goals. You are not just doing this for the sake of weight loss but also to help you remain accountable to your goals. When everyone is on board, they will make sure not to push junk food your way or involve you in conversations that will otherwise weigh you down.

Finally, if you walk downtown, you will notice that there are several creative markets selling special low-carb diets. It is easy to fall for these markets. While you need to eat low-carb diets to successfully lose weight, the most practical way how is to load on real food. This way, you will lose weight sustainably.

Chapter 11 The best weight-loss friendly foods

It is true that not all calories are created the same. One thing you must realize is that different foods will go through different metabolic pathways once they get into the body. The truth is that they can vary in the effect they have on your hunger, the number of calories, and hormones.

Some of the weight-loss friendly foods I ate on my weight loss program include;

Whole eggs

One of the misconceptions that people have had for years is that eggs are really high in cholesterol. Today, we know that eggs are making such a comeback. Even though consumption of high quantities of eggs has been shown to cause an increase in the levels of bad LDL cholesterol, they are still considered one of the best foods for weight loss. They are not only loaded with proteins but also good fats, making them satiating.

According to one study conducted in over 30 overweight and obese women who ate eggs for breakfast, there was a significant increase in the feelings of satiety. In fact, the research participants ate less for the next 36 hours.

The truth is, eggs are loaded with nutrients, and by including them into your diet plan, you not only get the nutrients you need on a calorie-restricted diet but also shed those extra pounds.

Leafy greens

These include such greens as spinach, swiss chards, kales, collards, and many others. the thing I love most about leafy greens is the fact that they have a wide range of properties that promote weight loss. For instance, they are low in carbs and calories, while at the same time are loaded with fiber.

According to experts, eating leafy greens is one of the best ways to increase the volume of your meals without necessarily packing on more calories. Research also indicates that when you load up on foods that are low energy density – like leafy greens – you end up consuming fewer calories at the end of the day. These greens are loaded with vitamins, minerals, and antioxidants that help the body in fat burning.

Salmon

Oh, there is nothing as filling like fatty fish – salmon and the rest. They are nutritious and satisfying while keeping you full for hours with just a few calories. Salmons are packed with high-quality proteins and healthy fats. They also have a significant amount of iodine, which plays an important role in the proper functioning of the thyroid. This, in turn, ensures that the rate of metabolism is at its optimal.

Salmons are also packed with omega-3-fatty acids, which lower inflammations – something that has been associated with lowering the risk of metabolic diseases and obesity.

Other types of fatty fishes you can eat in place of salmons include herring, mackerel, sardines, and trout.

Cruciferous veggies

These are cabbages, broccoli, Brussel sprouts, and cauliflower. Just like most veggies, these cruciferous veggies are loaded with fiber, making them incredibly satisfying. They also have been shown to contain a decent amount of proteins. While the level of proteins here is not as high as in animal foods or legumes, they are high-quality proteins most veggies do not have.

Their fiber, protein, and low-energy density makes these veggies the perfect foods for weight loss. They are also loaded with nutrients that have cancer-fighting substances, hence improves your overall health.

Fish

This is another low-calorie food that is loaded with high-quality protein. The fact that it is lean fish simply means that it is low in fat. This is one of the foods that has been shown to gain popularity among bodybuilders and fitness models on a cut. To ensure that you keep your total calories and fat as low as possible while increasing your protein intake, fill your plate with grilled Fish!

Beans and legumes

There are beans and legumes that have been shown to be beneficial to weight loss. These are black beans, lentils, and kidney beans, among others. They are not only high in fiber and protein, which contributes to satiety but also contain resistant starch.

Unfortunately, many people have difficulties tolerating legumes and hence the need to prepare them well.

Soups

As we have already mentioned, foods that are low-energy-density have a tendency of helping people eat fewer calories. The reason is that these kinds of foods contain lots of water – such as fruits and veggies. However, what I love most about them is that you can use them in making soups.

According to research, the same foods that can be turned and eaten as soup are filling and lead to the consumption of considerably fewer calories. The trick is to ensure that you are not adding too much fat in your soup – like cream and coconut milk – as these tend to increase your caloric intake.

Cottage cheese

One thing we all know about dairy products is that they are high in protein content. The best ones are cottage cheeses, which are loaded with proteins and very few carbs as well as little fat. If you want to boost your protein intake, cottage cheese is the way to go!

They are satisfying and makes you full for longer on relatively fewer calories. They are also rich in calcium, which has been attributed to fat burning. Other variants of this include the skyr and Greek Yoghurt.

Avocados

This is a unique fruit that should never miss in your plate. Unlike other fruits, avocados are low in carbs and yet packed with healthy fats. They are loaded with monounsaturated oleic acid, which is quite similar to the ones found in olive oil.

They also contain fiber and water, making them less energy-dense. You can use them to make veggie salads. Research shows that their fat content increases carotenoid antioxidant absorption from the veggies by 15-folds. Avocados are also packed with potassium and fiber.

Apple cider vinegar

Do you love using apple cider vinegar in making your dressings or vinaigrettes? Well, don't stop! This is one of the most popular additions in the natural health community. Research shows that adding this to your diet plan is useful for weight loss. They can increase feelings of satiety ad make you eat as little as 300 calories less than normal for the rest of the day. In fact, one study shows that the consumption of apple cider vinegar in their meals lowers 2.6-3.7 pounds of weight.

This has also been shown to lower the blood sugar spikes that often happen after meals, which goes a long way in bolstering your overall wellbeing in the long haul.

Nuts

Although they are high in fat, nuts are not fattening as most people think. According to research studies, eating nuts play an important role in boosting metabolic health and promoting weight loss. In fact, research studies demonstrate that people who eat nuts are often healthier and leaner compared to those who don't.

The trick here is to eat your nuts in moderation. If you go overboard, you end up with more calories than you need, hence stalling your weight loss.

Whole grains

For several years, cereal grains have had a bad reputation. However, not all cereals are bad for you because there are others that are definitely healthy. Whole grains are packed with fiber and a decent amount of proteins. Some of these whole grains include oats and quinoa.

One thing I love most about oats is that they are rich in bet-glucans, which is a soluble fiber that is not only feeling but also boosts metabolic health significantly. On the other hand, brown rice contains resistant starch, especially when they are cooked and allowed to cool after.

That said, note that refined grains are not a healthy choice for your weight loss goals. They are not only fattening but also harmful to your health and wellbeing. Therefore, if you are on a low-carb diet, try as much as you can to keep off grains because they are high carbs. However, there is nothing wrong with whole grains as long as you can tolerate them.

Chili pepper

This is one of the foods that never lacks in my food. If there is no chilling, the food is tasteless – but that is just me. Not everyone appreciates hot pepper in their food. The thing with chili pepper is that it plays an important role in promoting weight loss. It is packed with capsaicin, which lowers appetite and boosts fat burning. If you look keenly, you will realize that it is one of the ingredients used in most weight loss supplements.

According to one study, eating at least a gram of red chili pepper in a meal lowers appetite and boosts fat burning, especially in people who don't eat peppers regularly. However, there was really no effect on people who were used to eating spicy foods regularly. This indicates that certain tolerance levels could be built.

Chia seeds

This is one of the most nutritious foods on planet earth. I don't know about you, but chia seeds never miss in my cereal, not to mention other foods. In an ounce, at least 11 grams is fiber! This simply makes chia seeds low-carb friendly and the best source of fiber in the world, yet.

Because of its high fiber content, they are known to absorb up to 12 times of their weight in water, turning gel-like and expand in the stomach. With chia seeds, you can lower your appetite significantly and achieve your weight loss goals.

Chapter 12 Tips and tricks to make your journey successful

Hydrate

When you make water, your friend 24/7, makes it easier for you to hydrate as much as possible. Start from the time you get up by taking a glass or two of water and keep drinking periodically throughout the day. You should take at least 64-80 ounces of water daily. When your urine is clear, you know you are well hydrated. If not, keep taking it.

Give up on sodas

This also includes other diet varieties that are loaded with artificial sweeteners or sugars. When I first started my weight loss journey, I chose to take diet soda as a way of "spicing" things up. However, what I noticed is that each time I took them, they increased my sugar cravings and pushed me into making unhealthy diet choices.

You don't want that, so quit those sodas and sugar drinks.

Stay off carbs

You will be amazed at how fast your calories increase as you indulge in junk foods and high carb diets. Instead of going for taking outs, simply prepare a home-cooked meal with all the natural and carb-free ingredients. You will be amazed at how easy it is to transition from a diet loaded with processed foods and carbs to a clean meal plan.

Eat right

Load up with lean proteins, veggies, fresh fruits – preferably with fewer sugars – lean proteins, and low-fat dairy products. Stay off anything processed and with refined sugars and sodium. When you invest in eating nutrient-dense foods, you will lose weight with ease and feel better about it.

Go for small portions.

It is recommended that you go for three small portions of meals daily and at least 2-3 clean snacks. Instead of using a large plate, go for a smaller plate to ensure that your meal portions are in check. Each time you fill up a small plate, you get the illusion that you have eaten a lot already, and you stop it at that instead of going for an additional portion.

Read labels

It is necessary that before buying something at the grocery store or local supermarket, you check the labels and the ingredient list. If it has carbs, refined sugars, high sodium, or enriched white flour, leave it on the shelf.

Additionally, if you cannot pronounce each of the ingredients or don't even know what they are, just don't buy it.

If your goals are to lose weight and improve your wellbeing, the first tip is to get in the habit of reading labels so that you know exactly what you are putting into your body. You can also choose to skip the grocery aisles and stick to the perimeter of the store where you get fresh proteins, veggies, and fruits.

Chapter 13 FAQ's about weight loss

Should I weigh myself often?

It is best if you don't weigh yourself every day because the weight loss progress might not be reflected on the scales. However, you can weigh yourself at least once a week or twice a month to see real progress on the scale. People who successfully lose weight and sustainably keep it off weigh themselves occasionally at regular intervals. Doing it at least once a week plays an important role in building awareness.

That said, when you weight yourself and the numbers on the scale fluctuate from time, don't beat yourself up for it. Realize that weight changes by a couple of pounds over several days as the weight of water shifts.

Which fat should I cut back on to lose weight?

The shortest answer is saturated fats.

One thing you need to note – and according to the American dietary guidelines – is that less than 10% of your calories should come from saturated fats. When you don't eat a certain type of food, that does not necessarily translate to cutting on calories. The truth is that fat can help keep you stay fuller for longer, which lowers the risk of overeating.

Remember, your body needs dietary fat to function well. Therefore, instead of loading up on processed foods and butter, replace them with healthy polyunsaturated and monounsaturated fats – like cold-water fish, avocados, olive oil, nuts, and tofu. While lowering your intake of saturated fat is not a magic pill for weight loss. However, it plays a key role in improving your overall health and wellbeing.

To lose weight, should I drink plenty of water before meals?

It is true that drinking water before meals help fill you up so that you eat less. According to research studies, adults who drink at least 2 cups of water before eating their meals lose more weight compared to those who don't. That said, water plays an important role in helping keep you hydrated, and when your kidneys are actively moving water through the body, your water weight gets lower.

If you eat too much during lunch, should you starve during dinner?

If you are on a weight loss journey, it is best if you don't skip meals even in the event that you eat too much during lunch or any other meal, for that matter. The danger in skipping meals is that you risk becoming very hungry and be more apt to overeating or, even worse, indulging in junk foods. When this happens, your day's caloric intake goes potentially higher than you planned for.

Additionally, when you skip meals, you are less energized, and that lowers your likelihood of working out – which is key to successful and sustainable weight loss. Therefore, the best trick is to ensure that you have small, nutritious meals and snacks packed in between meals to help you stay full until the next meal, hence allowing you to lose more weight.

Remember, breakfast is the key to losing weight sustainably. Therefore, ensure that you faithfully take your breakfast to stay leaner and start the day off right.

During meals, how long should I take before being full?

It should take approximately 15-20 minutes. The key here is to ensure that you eat slowly especially if you want to achieve your weight loss goals. Research shows that there is a lag between when the food arrives in the mouth to the time when the brain registers your tummy is full. As you eat and pace yourself in between bites, you allow the brain more time to register when the stomach is full.

One study showed that women who were urged to take slow bites of low caloric foods during meal times drank plenty of water compared to those who ate quickly.

Should I plan every meal to lose weight?

That is right!

One thing you must note is that being spontaneous works for many activities, but not when it comes to eating. According to weight loss experts, it is best if you plan your meals and snacks to ensure that they are well suited for a balanced diet plan. If you don't have a good meal plan, you risk picking anything and everything you can find on the pantry shelves or in the fridge.

Should I keep a food diary?

Keeping a food diary goes a long way in ensuring that you not only keep track of what you eat but also double your weight loss according to one study. The good thing about journaling about food is that it makes you aware of how much you are eating and allows you to fix any bad eating habits you might have. It also keeps you more accountable so that you think through your meals before you take a bite. I use my fitnesspal app. It's very good.

Which carbs should I avoid to lose weight?

While carbs are generally not good for your body, the worst kind are those derived from processed foods. Avoid anything made and processed in a factory.Although low-carb diets have gained lots of popularity over the past years, you must realize that your body requires a few carbs for fuel. The healthy thing to do is ditch carbs from sugar-filled foods like junk foods, sodas, and animal fats. Instead, it is advisable that you load up on carbs derived from fruits, whole grains, and dark leafy veggies.

One Last Word

Indeed, weight loss is achievable.

If you thought that weight loss is unattainable, I believe this book has shown you how you can sustainably shed off those extra pounds, keep them off, and improve your diabetes condition once and for all. I have done it, and it's very easy under expert guidance. Just stay on course for the first fourteen days, and within 90 days, your habits and lifestyle will change.

This is the time to embark on a weight loss journey to a slimmer, fitter, and healthier version of you. Today is the day to begin your transformation to a healthy weight loss. This book will help you understand that good-for-you weight loss has nothing to do with yo-yo dieting! You will understand that weight loss is a good way for your body to function well and empower you to achieve long-term success.

You cannot transform your body all at once. That can be a recipe for disaster. The best trick is to set small but realistic goals you can work towards achieving them. You can start by taking a walk around the block at least four times a week instead of doing it every day.

If you do that, then these goals will soon become habits, and you can move on to the next objective. This will make you feel a sense of accomplishment, even as you progress with your weight loss goals. Remember, setbacks happen to all of us. So, don't let them discourage you from giving up!

There is also no such thing as a special diet exclusively for people with diabetes. While there is a wide range of ways to lose weight, there is no one-size-fits-all kind of diet. You must start by finding a way to eat fewer calories than you need. Find foods that are healthy for you and that promote weight loss. They must be whole foods like lean meats, veggies, fish, legumes, fruits, seeds, and nuts. If you couple your healthy food choices with moderate and regular workouts, you will not only achieve your weight loss goals but also pave the way for a healthy life. Remember that your health is your wealth!

The other trick to weight loss can be achieved through intermittent fasting. Remember, intermittent fasting is not a diet! Think of it as a timed- approach to eating. Unlike other dietary plans you know of that restrict caloric intake and the sources thereof, this approach does not specify the kind of food you should eat or avoid. It involves cycling between eating and fasting periods.

Even though intermittent fasting was at the forefront of helping me lose weight, one thing you must realize is that it is not sustainable for everyone. When getting started, most people find it challenging to eat during short intervals every day or even alternating between days of non-eating and eating.

The best trick here is to ensure that you are eating to your fill during eating windows. Don't overstuff yourself with food during eating windows. With a proper meal plan in place, you will ensure that you don't skip meals whenever you are busy or thrown off schedule and that when you eat, you get the required portion – nothing less, nothing more – just enough!

Also, choose an intermittent fasting plan that best suits your lifestyle. You want a plan you can maintain for the long haul. Also, consult with your dietitian to ensure that the decision you make is based on a proper assessment of your lifestyle and dietary requirements.

Moreover, you don't have to grind out hours of your day trying to burn fats. The main reason is that you have HIIT – High-intensity interval training – that will help you achieve your cardio fitness in just a short time. HIIT is often referred to as an all-out workout that requires exhaustive physical effort just for a short duration. In other instances, it is active recovery.

One thing you must remember is that when done well, HIIT can be a saving cardio grace. It has the potential of delivering a lot of the results you are looking for – elevated heart rate, fat burning, improved lung capacity, and pushing you to sweat. You can achieve all these and more in just a fraction of time, hence considered a very useful workout for people who prefer not to spend all day in the gym. The key here is the intensity.

You cannot achieve your weight loss goals without shifting your mindset for weight loss. Realize that you cannot change your weight from the outside before you get your inner resolve and intention aligned with your goals. Don't try to lose weight by wanting to "fix" yourself. It is this mentality that makes people jump into exercise and diet plans out of self-deprecation, while they still call themselves "fat" and feel less than they are all together.

Losing weight is not about focusing the mind on quick fixes. It is setting the mind on sustainability and wellbeing. Your mindset should be that you are doing this to improve your health, enjoyment, and longer life.

What helped me lose weight is simple; a very strict, no-carb diet. All I had was salads and proteins – veggies, boiled eggs, fish, and meat, among others.

Today, take up the challenge and do whatever it takes to ensure that your health is back on track. There are no cheat days here. No alcohol. These are the things that played an important role in helping me lose weight fast and sustainably.

So, what are you still waiting for?

Start your weight loss journey and achieve your goals and improve your wellbeing.

Best wishes!

Resources

1. Nitric Oxide Dump

   https://youtu.be/QgfoByLYdYc

2. Farmers Walk

   https://youtu.be/KlmtWHC61nk

3. HIIT Workout

   https://www.youtube.com/watch?v=H83DhoCPU

www.ingramcontent.com/pod-product-compliance
Lightning Source LLC
Chambersburg PA
CBHW071217240726

48654CB00009B/819